Atlas of
Laparoscopic Colon Surgery

Atlas of
Laparoscopic Colon Surgery

Moises Jacobs, M.D.

Clinical Assistant Professor of Surgery, Department of Surgery,
University of Miami School of Medicine; International Medical Director,
Laparoscopic Surgery Center, Baptist Hospital of Miami,
Miami, Florida

Gustavo Plasencia, M.D.

Clinical Professor of Surgery, Department of Surgery,
University of Miami School of Medicine,
Miami, Florida

Philip F. Caushaj, M.D.

Associate Professor of Surgery and Program Director,
Laparoscopy and Surgical Endoscopy, University of Massachusetts
Medical School; Chairman, Department of Surgery,
The Medical Center of Central Massachusetts,
Worcester, Massachusetts

with 140 illustrations

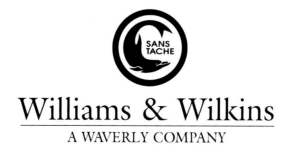

Williams & Wilkins

A WAVERLY COMPANY

BALTIMORE • PHILADELPHIA • LONDON • PARIS • BANGKOK
BUENOS AIRES • HONG KONG • MUNICH • SYDNEY • TOKYO • WROCLAW

Editor: Carroll C. Cann
Production Coordinator: Peter J. Carley
Typesetter: The Type House
Printer: Mandarin Offset
Binder: Mandarin Offset

351 West Camden Street
Baltimore, Maryland 21201-2436   USA

Rose Tree Corporate Center
1400 North Providence Road
Building II, Suite 5025
Media, Pennsylvania 19063-2043   USA

Accurate indications, adverse reactions and dosage schedules for drugs are provided in this book, but it is possible that they may change. The reader is urged to review the package information data of the manufacturers of the medications mentioned.

Printed in Hong Kong

Library of Congress Cataloging-in-Publication Data

Jacobs, Moises.
    Atlas of laparoscopic colon surgery / Moises Jacobs, Gustavo
Plasencia, Philip F. Caushaj.
        p.   cm.
    Includes bibliographical references and index.
    ISBN 0-683-30032-6
    1. Colon (Anatomy)—Endoscopic surgery.   2. Laparoscopic surgery.
I. Plasencia, Gustavo.   II. Caushaj, Philip F.   III. Title.
    [DNLM: 1. Colon—surgery.   2. Surgery, Laparoscopic—methods.
3. Colectomy—methods.   WI 520 J17a 1996]
RD544.J33   1996
617.5′547—dc20
DNLM/DLC
for Library of Congress   96-15262
                                                                CIP

The publishers have made every effort to trace the copyright holders for borrowed material. If they have inadvertently overlooked any, they will be pleased to make the necessary arrangements at the first sopportunity.

To purchase additional copies of this book, call our customer service department at **(800) 638-0672** or fax orders to **(800) 447-8438.** For other book services, including chapter reprints and large quantity sales, ask for the Special Sales department.

Canadian customers should call **(800) 268-4178** or fax **(905) 470-6780.** For all other calls originating outside of the United States, please call **(410) 528-4223** or fax us at **(410) 528-8550.**

Visit Williams & Wilkins on the Internet: **http://www.wwilkins.com** or contact our customer service department at **custserv@wwilkins.com.** Williams & Wilkins customer service representatives are available from 8:30 am to 6:00 pm, EST, Monday through Friday, for telephone access.

95   96   97   98   99
1   2   3   4   5   6   7   8   9   10

To

Family and friends
for their guidance and support
throughout our lives and for always being
there when we needed them

M.J. and *G.P.*
Miami, Florida

My wife, **Shpresa,**
whose love and support have made everything
possible and worthwhile; my children, **Kate** and **Sam,**
whose love fills my life; my mother, **Virginia,** sister, **Donika,** and
late father, **Sam,** whose unconditional love and support
are my personal strength; **Nena, Liri,** and **Bob,**
whose love has brightened my life

P.F.C.
Worcester, Massachusetts

Contributors

Philip F. Caushaj, M.D.
Associate Professor of Surgery and Program Director, Laparoscopy and Surgical Endoscopy, University of Massachusetts Medical School; Chairman, Department of Surgery, The Medical Center of Central Massachusetts, Worcester, Massachusetts

Timothy C. Counihan, M.D.
Chief Resident, University of Massachusetts Coordinated Surgical Residency Program, Worcester, Massachusetts

Morris Franklin, M.D.
Clinical Professor of Surgery, University of Texas Health Sciences Center; Director, Texas Endosurgery Institute, San Antonio, Texas

W. Peter Geis, M.D.
Clinical Professor of Surgery, University of Chicago, Chicago, Illinois; Director, Minimally Invasive Surgery Training Institute, Department of Surgery, St. Joseph Hospital, Baltimore, Mayland

Rene F. Hartmann, M.D.
Assistant Professor of Clinical Surgery; Chief, Department of Colon and Rectal Surgery, University of Miami, Miami, Florida

Moises Jacobs, M.D.
Clinical Assistant Professor of Surgery, Department of Surgery, University of Miami School of Medicine; International Medical Director, Laparoscopic Surgery Center, Baptist Hospital of Miami, Miami, Florida

Sergio W. Larach, M.D.
Clinical Associate Professor, Department of Surgery, University of Florida College of Medicine, Orlando, Florida; Program Director, Colon and Rectal Fellowship at Orlando Regional Medical Center, Orlando, Florida

Daniel T. Martin, M.D.
Assistant Professor, Department of Surgery, University of New Mexico School of Medicine, Albuquerque, New Mexico

Joseph P. McDermott, M.D.
Surgical Endoscopy Fellow, Medical Center of Central Massachusetts, Worcester, Massachusetts

Gustavo Plasencia, M.D.
Clinical Professor of Surgery, Department of Surgery, University of Miami School of Medicine, Miami, Florida

Manuel Viamonte III, M.D.
Clinical Assistant Professor, Department of Surgery, University of Miami School of Medicine, Miami, Florida

Karl A. Zucker, M.D.
Professor of Surgery, Department of Surgery, University of New Mexico School of Medicine, Albuquerque, New Mexico

Foreword

One of the most gratifying aspects in the recent history of surgery has been the unexpected close relationships that have developed among the pioneers of laparoscopic surgery. These friendships would not have been possible had surgery not taken a major change of course. It is with great pleasure that I recommend to you this text on laparoscopic colon surgery by three such pioneers.

As we progress toward the twenty-first century, the surgical movement of laparoscopy continues to grow exponentially. This outgrowth of knowledge is based on the solid foundations of surgeons who have spent years perfecting the open techniques in their areas of expertise. Additionally, they have been willing to delve into a new way of thinking as well as a new way of practicing their surgical skills in the operating suite.

The authors of *Atlas of Laparoscopic Colon Surgery* provide comprehensive coverage of minimally invasive colon surgery based on the largest reported series to date in the surgical literature. The authors' representation of these techniques and results is a welcome addition to the laparoscopic surgeon's library of reference material.

Colon surgery, unlike other procedures, depends on specimen retrieval, may involve other organs, and in essence requires that one must have an in-depth knowledge of all quadrants of the abdomen. Success in minimally invasive colon surgery depends on adherence to the fundamentals of surgery, including a solid knowledge of laparoscopy, detailed understanding of anatomy, skill in laparoscopic suturing, and most important, patience.

As technology improves and large specimens are retrieved, what is laparoscopically assisted colon surgery today will become totally laparoscopic in the future. State of the art is carefully presented in this text for the operating surgeon who wishes to become proficient in laparoscopic colon surgery. Clinical caveats at the end of each chapter provide the reader with experience-born "tips of the trade" the surgeon will find invaluable.

I congratulate Drs. Moises Jacobs, Gustavo Plasencia, and Philip F. Caushaj on their pioneering contribution to the laparoscopic surgical literature.

J. Barry McKernan, M.D.
Professor of Surgery, Emory University and
the Medical College of Georgia

Preface

---∎---

Surgery, indeed all of medicine, is currently undergoing significant socioeconomic paradigm shifts. The advent and popularity of minimally invasive techniques have challenged the historical tenets and scientific foundations of surgical procedures that, until recently, had been unchanged and unchallenged by alternatives. Advances of the last 40 years have forced critical reappraisal of perioperative management as well as minor modifications to surgical procedures. Classic debates in general and colorectal surgery over the last two decades have focused on such issues as when and whether to use drains, the rationale for using or omitting nasogastric tubes, and the best methods for closing the abdominal wall.

The explosion ignited by the introduction and proliferation of laparoscopic cholecystectomy has propelled the laparoscopic approach to the forefront as the procedure of choice and the standard of care for most symptomatic biliary tract disorders. Although the debate still rages as to whether selective versus routine intraoperative cholangiography is indicated or what the role is for draining the gallbladder fossa, logarithmic changes have altered the perioperative management of these patients as well as the clinical outcomes.

This clinical shift of paradigms has occurred at a time when outcome analysis and costs are under extreme scrutiny. While laparoscopic approaches to disorders of the foregut have also been rapidly gaining acceptance internationally, this has not been the case for laparoscopic approaches for treatment of disorders of the colon and rectum. Dramatic reports of trocar site tumor implantation have raised significant concerns in the surgical community as to whether this technologic advance should be offered as the primary treatment for colorectal malignancies, the most common indication for colorectal surgery in Western nations. We used laparoscopic approaches for such malignancies relatively early in our combined laparoscopic colorectal experience. We did so separately, employing the basic surgical principles that we believe are necessary to protect our patients. First, we used laparoscopic procedures for other indications: laparoscopic cholecystectomy, appendectomy, and fundoplication were routine in our clinical practices. Second, and most important, we performed the same oncologic operation that we had previously performed using conventional techniques, steadfastly adhering to the principles we firmly believe in. When we thought there was a danger that an oncologic principle might be violated, the procedure was converted to an open approach and we completed our standard procedure. These conversions are not viewed as failures but as expressions of good judgment and of our concern for our patients' well-being.

As we have traveled extensively, sharing our experience with our colleagues throughout the world, we have had many requests to reduce to writing our technical approaches to laparoscopic colorectal surgery. The most significant lesson we have gleaned from our extensive and early experience is the technically demanding nature of the laparoscopic technique for disorders of the colon and rectum. Indeed, the only significant reason that this minimally invasive approach to colorectal surgery has not been widely adapted, as have procedures for the gallbladder and disorders of the foregut, is not the specter of inadequacy of the oncologic surgery but the reality that the techniques necessary for successful laparoscopic colorectal surgery are difficult to learn. We hope that by sharing our approach we may help our colleagues to develop their skills and thus be able to offer their patients the acknowledged benefits of minimally invasive surgery, such as reduced morbidity, an earlier return to normal activity, and improved functional outcomes.

Unlike other procedures mastered during our residencies and fellowships, there were no books to guide us through these approaches to laparoscopic colorectal surgery. Many colleagues throughout the world freely shared information, tips, and advice; the direct exchange of ideas sometimes actually precedes publication in today's global community! There have been many surgeons who helped us develop our skills and to whom we are extremely grateful. Some have been pioneers in laparoscopic surgery and, in addition to being our friends, have most generously shared their experience with us. You may recognize the thread of their thoughts throughout this book. If the ideas presented herein are worthy, please offer the credit to these intrepid individuals. If the concepts discussed in these pages do not meet your expectations, we have failed to deliver their message. To Morris Franklin, J. Barry McKernan, W. Peter Geis, Robert Beart, John Coller, John Murray, James Fleshman, Anne Mosenthal, and many others too numerous to list, we express our humble gratitude.

We have been guided throughout the publishing process by the dauntless efforts and vision of our editor, Beth Campbell, and publisher, Karen Berger, of Quality Medical Publishing. Suzanne Wakefield cajoled and nudged until all the elements came together, and Judy Bamert rendered the whole in lucid page layouts. Medical illustrator Floyd Hosmer is to be commended for his line drawings that illustrate each step of these procedures. The perspective of these drawings replicates the view through the laparoscope, including the effects of gravity on internal organs.

We hope this *Atlas of Laparoscopic Colon Surgery* will serve as a tool for developing and refining the laparoscopic approach for disorders of the colon and rectum. Inevitably, in due course this book will be outdated by the continuing advances in laparoscopic surgery. As certain as we are that there will be some who find fault with our message, we are equally certain that the basic principles of minimally invasive colorectal surgery will survive the test of time.

Moises Jacobs
Gustavo Plasencia
Philip F. Caushaj

Contents

Part One

PRINCIPLES

1

The Evolution of Laparoscopic General Surgery

Joseph P. McDermott ▪ Philip F. Caushaj

Although laparoscopic surgery is often perceived as a recent surgical advance, in actuality laparoscopic approaches have been used for almost a century. Modern laparoscopy is safer, faster, and easier than earlier versions, reflecting the marriage of technology and biomedical ingenuity that have revitalized this surgical approach and thrust laparoscopic surgery to the forefront of modern medicine. It remains to be seen whether laparoscopic technique will become a staple of surgical practice or will eventually return to obscurity, to be remembered as a passing fad of the late twentieth century. In the interim, surgeons are availing themselves of the increasingly sophisticated technology being developed in an attempt to offer the best possible care for their patients.

The pioneers in the field have been drawn from many different disciplines: physicians, scientists, engineers, and surgeons have all made landmark contributions to the advancement of laparoscopy. Gynecologists were among the first to recognize the value of laparoscopy; general surgeons have only recently taken notice of the advantages of minimally invasive technique.

The Early Years: Physician Pioneers and a New Technology

In 1901 Ott, from Petrograd, Russia reported examining the abdominal cavity of patients through a small abdominal or pelvic incision. He held the incision open with a speculum and used a reflecting head mirror and an incandescent light to view the abdominal contents. Although similar to a mini-laparotomy rather than to laparoscopy, this *ventroscopy* permitted accurate diagnosis of many common diseases of the day. The earliest published report of laparoscopy was by Kelling of Dresden, Germany in 1902. With a procedure he called *koelioskopie* (celioscopy), he insufflated the peritoneal cavity of a dog with air, then inspected it using a cystoscope. These early attempts to "examine the flank" laid the foundation for the development of modern laparoscopy.

The first publication of a major series of laparoscopies in humans came in 1911. Swedish physician Jacobaeus, in his series of 72 patients, described performing laparoscopy as well as thoracoscopy. He reported the laparoscopic identification of syphilis, tuberculosis, cirrhosis, and malignancy.

The first report of laparoscopy in the United States was also published in 1911. Bertram M. Bernheim from Johns Hopkins University drew on information published by Jacobaeus in 1910 to perform his first laparoscopic procedure. Although his reported experience consisted of only two patients, it signaled the emigration of laparoscopic technique from Europe to America.

Despite multiple reports of successful laparoscopic operations performed during the first quarter of this century, laparoscopic technique was not widely embraced by physicians and surgeons. The technology and instrumentation needed to perform safe and easy laparoscopy had not yet been developed, and drawbacks such as the small field of vision, poor illumination, and risk of thermal injury from the light source proved to be limiting factors.

Although Kelling and others reported creation of a pneumoperitoneum using a needle and filtered air, many laparoscopists introduced their trocars and laparoscopes (usually modified cystoscopes) directly into the peritoneal cavity to avoid injury from the insufflation needle and the possible side effects associated with a pneumoperitoneum. Most physicians reserved laparoscopy for patients with gross ascites: the ascites would be drained and the peritoneal cavity reexpanded with filtered air. The rapid expansion of the abdomen in the absence of ascites was felt to be dangerous. Goetz suggested the use of a safety needle for creation of a pneumoperitoneum in 1918; however, it was not until Veress developed his version of a spring-loaded safety needle in 1938 that this technique became popular.

In 1924, Zollikofer of Switzerland proposed using carbon dioxide rather than the standard filtered air to develop the pneumoperitoneum, since carbon dioxide was more easily absorbed. He stated that "gaseous expansion of the abdomen is harmless and tolerated only by patients in whom emptying of the ascitic fluid is possible; such distention causes reflex action of the vagus on the heart. Therefore, pathological changes of the gallbladder, appendix, and adnexa as a rule will not be objects of the laparoscopic method."

In the first half of this century, many surgeons in the United States remained skeptical about laparoscopy. Other physicians were more impressed with the potential of this technology. J.C. Ruddock, an internist, published a report in 1937 of 500 successful *peritoneoscopies,* including 39 biopsies. Ironically, he chose a major surgical journal as his forum. Despite this wake-up call to the surgical community, it would be many more decades before significant interest would be aroused in the surgical community.

Technologic Advances

In 1966 a British optical physicist named Hopkins developed a rod-lens system for the laparoscope that greatly improved its brightness and clarity. This rod-lens system, coupled with the newly developed fiberoptic "cold" light source, proved to be one of the greatest advancements in the field of laparoscopic surgery. Laparoscopic technology was becoming increasingly sophisticated and sensitive, and in the process was attracting the attention of surgeons around the world, most notably in gynecologic surgery.

As the technical problems of laparoscopy were slowly being overcome, surgeons attempted to do more than just view and biopsy the abdominal and pelvic organs. These efforts to expand laparoscopic applications were prompted by the introduction of technologic innovations. Semm of Kiel, Germany developed an automatic insufflation device that monitored abdominal pressure and gas flow. The machine is still used today with few modifications from the original version.

Hasson, in 1974, developed a trocar for open laparoscopy. This trocar was placed directly into the abdominal cavity through a small incision, and then the pneumoperitoneum was created by pumping carbon dioxide through the trocar. This obviated the need for a blind puncture by an insufflation needle, thus decreasing the risk of visceral and retroperitoneal injuries during needle insertion and making reoperative laparoscopy safer.

In the mid-1980s the development of computer chip television camera technology allowed the laparoscopic image to be projected onto a monitor, making surgical assistance and laparoscopic training easier and faster. Procedures could be recorded on a video tape for reviewing and teaching the technique. Before this technologic breakthrough, the surgeon and assistant viewed the laparoscopic field through image-splitting laparoscopic devices, although illumination of the field was often compromised.

As technology improved, increasing numbers of reports of therapeutic laparoscopic procedures appeared in the literature. DeKok described the first laparoscopically assisted appendectomy in 1977. Only 1 year later, Frimberg performed a cholecystotomy using the laparoscopic technique. Semm is credited with performing the first completely laparoscopic appendectomy in 1983. In what would become the start of the laparoscopic general surgery explosion, Mouret performed the first laparoscopic cholecystectomy on a human in 1987 in Lyon, France.

The Laparoscopic Explosion

One year after Mouret's initial laparoscopic cholecystectomy, McKernan and Saye repeated the procedure in the United States. Reddick and Olsen from Nashville, Tennessee collaborated with McKernan and Saye to publish the first clinical report in the English literature on laparoscopic cholecystectomy in 1989.

Since these first published reports, the popularity of the laparoscopic technique has grown exponentially. Laparoscopic cholecystectomy has surpassed open cholecystectomy as the standard for gallbladder removal. This procedure has proved to be less painful, quicker, and more cost effective than the standard technique. By 1993 Deziel et al. were able to compile a survey analyzing 77,604 laparoscopic cholecystectomies performed in the United States. Corroborating smaller studies, they showed that the overall morbidity and mortality of laparoscopic cholecystectomy was comparable with or lower than that of open cholecystectomy, although there was a slightly higher rate of common bile duct injury.

With the apparent success of laparoscopic cholecystectomy, surgeons rapidly applied this technique to other common general surgical procedures, such as supraduodenal exploration of the common bile duct and advanced biliary surgery.

One of the first reports of laparoscopic inguinal herniorrhaphy was by Ger et al. in 1989. Although this report was of a canine model, the idea was quickly applied to humans. However, the exact role of the laparoscopic approach in hernia repair is still being evaluated. The initial excitement has been tempered by reports of unusual and standard complications, including recurrence of hernia. The role of this new technology in the treatment of inguinal hernias needs further investigation.

Laparoscopic appendectomy has gained in popularity as the success of the laparoscopic cholecystectomy has become obvious. Although Semm first described his laparoscopic appendectomy 4 years before Mouret performed the first laparoscopic cholecystectomy, prospective trials comparing laparoscopic and open appendectomy are just now beginning to be published. Although the patient's hospital stay is usually shorter when laparoscopic technique is used, this is often offset by a higher total cost of hospitalization. Selective use of the laparoscope in the diagnosis and treatment of appendiceal disease may prove to be most beneficial and cost effective.

Gastric surgery is gaining a revitalized popularity as the laparoscopic approach is being applied to procedures for gastroesophageal reflux and peptic ulcer disease. Initial results of these laparoscopic procedures are promising, but as with most new techniques, long-term results must be awaited.

Laparoscopic technique is being applied to all aspects of general surgery. Splenectomy, adrenalectomy, and even laparoscopically assisted pancreaticoduodenectomy are under investigation. The value of the laparoscopic technique in various types of operations will be fully understood only after trials are completed comparing this technique with standard operations.

Laparoscopic colon surgery is also being performed as an alternative to the open approach. In 1990 Jacobs et al. performed the first laparoscopically assisted colectomy (personal communication, 1994). By 1991 there were at least half a dozen reports of laparoscopic colon resections published in the English literature. The laparoscopic technique is being used for the treatment of both benign and malignant disorders, and prospective studies are underway to determine its safety and efficacy in these applications.

The Future of Laparoscopic Surgery

Technologic advances will continue to broaden the possible indications for laparoscopic surgery. New instrumentation will make complex surgical maneuvers easier. The development of a three-dimensional video system is being actively pursued and prototypes are being field evaluated. The surgeon's ability to operate in a three-dimensional field may increase the speed of surgery and decrease the difficulty of the surgeon's learning curve. At present the three-dimensional picture lacks the clarity of high-definition, two-dimensional video. As this problem is overcome, three-dimensional laparoscopy may prove to be a useful adjunct.

Indications for the use of laparoscopic surgery continue to expand and appear to be limited only by advances in technology and the ingenuity of surgeons. Yet the laparoscopic technique may not be appropriate for all types of surgery. Randomized, controlled trials to evaluate the safety and cost-effectiveness of the laparoscopic technique as compared with that of open surgery will decide the future of this surgical advancement.

Bibliography

A phase III prospective randomized trial comparing laparoscopic assisted colectomy versus standard colectomy for colon cancer—the intergroup trial: NCCTG, SWOG, CALBG. Rochester, Minn, 1993.

Bernheim BM. Organoscopy: Cystoscopy of the abdominal cavity. Ann Surg 53:764, 1911.

Cuschieri AE. Hiatal hernia and reflux esophagitis. In Hunter JG, Sackier JM, eds. Minimally Invasive Surgery. New York: McGraw-Hill, 1993.

Cuschieri AE. Laparoscopic vagotomy: Gimmick or reality. Surg Clin North Am 72:357, 1992.

DeKok H. A new technique for resecting the noninflamed, nonadhesive appendix through a mini-laparotomy with the aid of the laparoscope. Arch Chir Nederl 29:195-197, 1977.

Deziel DJ, Millikan KW, Economou SG, Doolas A, Ko ST, Airan MC. Complications of laparoscopic cholecystectomy: A national survey of 4,292 hospitals and analysis of 77,604 cases. Am J Surg 165:9, 1993.

Dubois F, Berthelot G, Levard H. Laparoscopic cholecystectomy: Historical perspective and personal experience. Surg Laparosc Endosc 1:525, 1991.

Ger R, Monroe K, Duvivier R, Mishrick A. Management of indirect hernias by laparoscopic closure of the neck of the sac. Am J Surg 159:370, 1990.

Goetze O. Die Rontgendiagnostik bei Gasgefullter Bauchhohle: Eine neue Methode. Munch Med Wochenschr 65:25, 1918.

Hasson HM. Open laparoscopy vs. closed laparoscopy: A comparison of complication rates. Adv Plann Parent 13:41-50, 1978.

Jacobaeus HC. Uber die Moglichkeit die Zystoskopie bei untersuchung seroser hohlungen anzuwenden. Munch Med Wochenschr 58:2090, 1910.

Jacobaeus HC. Ubersicht uber meine Erfahrungen mit der Laparothorakoskopie. Munch Med Wochenschr 57:2017, 1911.

Jacobs M, Verdeja JC, Goldstein HS. Laparoscopic choledocholithotomy. J Laparoendosc 1:79, 1991.

Katkhouda N, Mouiel J. A new surgical technique of treatment of chronic duodenal ulcer without laparotomy by videocoelioscopy. Am J Surg 161:361, 1991.

Kelling G. Ueber Oesophagoskopie, Gastroskopie und Koelioskopie. Munch Med Wochenschr 49:21, 1902.

MacFadyen B. Complications of laparoscopic herniorrhaphy [abst]. SAGES Symp 5:9, 1992.

Nadeau OE, Kampmeier OF. Endoscopy of the abdomen. Abdominoscopy: A preliminary study, including a summary of the literature and a description of the technique. Surg Gynecol Obstet 41:259, 1925.

Ott D. Illumination of the abdomen (ventroscopia) [Russian]. J Akush i Zhensk 15: Stellato T. History of laparoscopic surgery. Surg Clin North Am 72:997, 1992.

Reddick EJ, Olsen D, Daniell J, Saye W, McKernan B, Miller W, Hoback M. Laparoscopic laser cholecystectomy. Laser Med Surg News Adv 38, 1989.

Ruddock JC. Peritoneoscopy. Surg Gynecol Obstet 65:623, 1937.

Semm K. Atlas of Gynecologic Laparoscopy and Hysteroscopy. Philadelphia: WB Saunders, 1977.

Semm K. Endoscopic appendectomy. Endoscopy 15:59, 1983.

Semm K. Operative Manual for Endoscopic Abdominal Surgery. Chicago: Year Book Medical Publishers, 1977.

Stellato T. History of laparoscopic surgery. Surg Clin North Am 72:997, 1992.

Vallina VL, Velasco JM, McColloch CS. Laparoscopic versus conventional appendectomy. Ann Surg 218:685, 1993.

Veress J. Nues Instrument zur ausfuhrung von brust-oder Bauchpunktionen und Pneumothoraxbehandlung. Dtsch Med Wochenschr 41:1480, 1938.

Zucker KA, Reddick EJ, Bailey RW, eds. Surgical Laparoscopy. St. Louis: Quality Medical Publishing, 1991, p 13.

2

Fundamental Principles and Perioperative Management

Philip F. Caushaj ▪ Moises Jacobs ▪ Gustavo Plasencia

11

Although it may seem logical to assume that experience with laparoscopic cholecystectomy confers an inherent advantage when performing more advanced laparoscopic procedures, this is not necessarily the case. The premise that all surgeons are created equal in judgment or technical ability is not true for conventional open surgery or for laparoscopic surgery. The basics of laparoscopic cholecystectomy are easily learned and experience can be rapidly gained, with low morbidity; nevertheless, complications have occurred following relatively basic laparoscopic procedures, with serious consequences. Laparoscopic cholecystectomy is performed in one field with relatively stable trocar insertions.

Laparoscopic procedures performed for the colon and rectum are far more complex than those for the gallbladder. There are multiple and variable trocar sites, the bowel must be placed on traction to be mobilized, and the techniques for gaining and applying traction vary. The operative field is dynamic and must change as certain objectives have been achieved during the course of the operation.

Essential to the performance of these more advanced procedures is a grasp of the fundamentals of laparoscopic surgery. The fundamentals that are basic to advanced laparoscopy will be discussed in this chapter. The specific details of trocar location, monitor positioning, and of each operation will be discussed in subsequent chapters.

The Operating Room Team

Before initiating a laparoscopic colorectal surgery protocol, it is important to develop a laparoscopic team familiar with the necessary instrumentation and equipment. The ability to position Babcock clamps and bowel clamps atraumatically and ensure traction can prevent complications. There must be interactive coordination between the surgeon, the first assistant, and the camera operator. Appropriate degrees of traction and countertraction are necessary to minimize iatrogenic injury to the bowel and mesentery. The camera operator and surgeon must coordinate their efforts. For example, when bleeding occurs, the operative field must not change, since it may prove difficult to find the same exposure, which can force conversion of a salvagable laparoscopic procedure to an open one. We believe strongly that a decision to convert a laparoscopic procedure to an open approach is not a complication but the exercise of good surgical judgment.

Preoperative Considerations

The patient must be secured to the operating room table for all laparoscopic surgical procedures. We employ a bean bag ordinarily used for thoracic surgical procedures to maintain the patient's position. Patient positioning is an important part of the operation and should not be relegated to the most junior person in the operating room; this should be performed or supervised by the surgeon to ensure that the patient is appropriately positioned. It is vexing and time consuming to reposition the patient during a laparoscopic procedure, and such repositioning can often result in frank violations of sterile technique.

All necessary instrumentation for conversion to an open procedure should be in the operating room for advanced laparoscopic colon and rectal surgery. This will minimize the time required for conversion in the event of complications or life-threatening hemorrhage.

Establishing the Pneumoperitoneum

There are several methods for establishing a pneumoperitoneum. In subsequent chapters we will not describe this technique again but will assume that any surgeon comfortable enough to proceed with advanced laparoscopic surgery has mastered a technique for establishing a pneumoperitoneum. The most commonly performed are the percutaneous technique, with a Veress needle, and the Hasson open technique. The relative merits of either method are well described in the literature. The merits of the Hasson open technique include the ability to gain exposure of the peritoneal cavity directly and to minimize injuries that could result from blind insertion of the Veress needle and primary trocar. The relative disadvantages of this method are that it is time consuming and may not offer as complete a seal to minimize the potential for desufflation from the trocar site. Some surgical laparoscopists advocate using this technique in selected patients who have had previous surgical incisions.

We use the percutaneous Veress technique for establishing the pneumoperitoneum (Fig. 2-1). In our experience with more than 1000 laparoscopic procedures, we have not encountered an episode of iatrogenic injury to bowel or solid viscera. There has been abdominal wall bleeding secondary to placement of either the Veress needle or the primary trocar, but incidence has been less than 0.1%. When we encounter previous midline incisions, instead of approaching the Veress needle insertion through the umbilicus, we select an alternative location in the left upper quadrant. This area has been frequently used in our surgical endoscopy practice for placing percutaneous endoscopic gastrostomy tubes. Clinically, this location is relatively safe in a previously operated abdomen. Nonetheless, iatrogenic injuries to the colon or stomach can occur. These injuries may, if recognized early, be technically easier to repair than the occasional aortic or iliac vessel injury encountered through the midline.

Once the Veress needle or Hasson trocar is inserted, the pneumoperi-

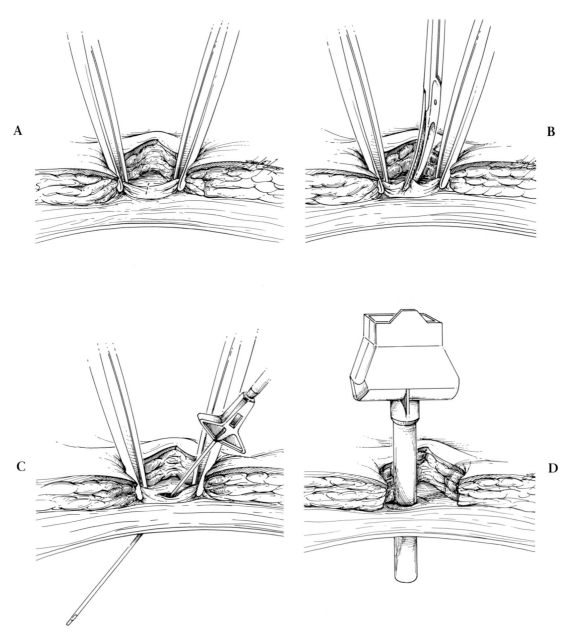

Fig. 2-1. A, A modified open approach combines some of the advantages of the standard closed and open techniques. Through a standard 10 to 15 mm incision, the fascia is grasped between Kocher clamps and elevated up to or near the skin incision. **B,** A small incision is made through the fascia to allow initial placement of the Veress needle. **C,** The insufflation needle is gently advanced through the peritoneum, and a clear but distinct "pop" can be felt by the surgeon. If intra-abdominal adhesions are present, the surgeon should meet resistance with the attempts at insertion. **D,** Once the abdomen is safely insufflated and the presence of underlying adhesions to the abdominal wall has been ruled out, a standard 10 mm port may then be inserted in a routine fashion. This will obviate the need for the use of a Hasson cannula. (From Bailey RW, Flowers JL, eds. Complications of Laparoscopic Surgery. St. Louis: Quality Medical Publishing, 1995.)

toneum is established with CO_2. The pressure limits are 10 to 15 mm Hg. The use of a high-flow insufflator with a capacity of 9.9 L/min is important. Multiple instrument changes as well as the movement of the trocars may lead to significant desufflation that may obscure the field of vision. Some laparoscopists advocate using two high-flow insufflators so that a trocar stopcock may be left open to desufflate the smoke that is often present following the application of cautery. The ability to distinguish a flow problem resulting from lack of CO_2 from desufflation caused by an open stopcock will allow a difficult technical operation to proceed as smoothly as possible. During each of the discussions of selected procedures, we will review the operating room setup: camera positions and their locations relative to the surgeons and assistants and patient position and trocar sites. Thus it is unnecessary to review these in great detail here. Gasless laparoscopy may offer an alternative in the future as more experience is gained with this modality. The potential benefits of gasless laparoscopy relate directly to the consequences of the use of CO_2: because this gas is rapidly absorbed, elevated P_{CO_2} and respiratory acidosis are associated with its use.

The safest approach to establishing a pneumoperitoneum is the technique that the surgeon is most comfortable with; neither technique reduces the possibility of iatrogenic injury to nil. Consequently, in obtaining informed consent one should review with the patient the potential for iatrogenic injuries; those that occur most frequently are of the bowel, bladder, blood vessels, and abdominal wall.

Diagnostic Laparoscopy

Before proceeding with secondary trocar placement, the surgeon must perform diagnostic laparoscopy. Exploration of the peritoneal cavity following a midline incision is surgical dogma, ingrained in every surgeon's thinking throughout his or her career. Not only is the palpable evaluation of structures necessary, but also a secondary visual inspection of the visceral surfaces must be performed. A clinical concern expressed regarding laparoscopic surgery is the loss of the ability to perform tactile evaluation of the abdominal contents. This may be overcome by manually exploring the abdomen during assisted procedures, or if the size of the surgeon's hand is sufficiently small, one can gain access through a small incision created to remove the specimen. The application of ultrasonography during diagnostic laparoscopy may offer an evaluation of the peritoneal cavity not previously encountered with manual palpation alone.

It is possible laparoscopically to inspect the peritoneal surfaces for abnormalities. Visualize the surfaces of the liver, aided by a 30-degree laparoscope, examine the small bowel from the ligament of Treitz to the terminal ileum, and inspect the gallbladder, bladder, and stomach. Although limited in actual practice, direct examination of the lesser sac is possible. Any pathologic abnormalities should be recorded and may alter the conduct of the operation. During an operation for malignancy, if there is any doubt about the stage of the tumor or any abnormality that would suggest a synchronous lesion, the surgeon should seriously consider converting to an open operation. Liver abnormalities can be laparoscopically biopsied, directly or with a Tru-Cut needle.

Conducting the Procedure

After diagnostic laparoscopy, secondary trocars can be placed. An excellent study by Yutzpe demonstrated that 22% of iatrogenic injuries related to needle or trocar insertion occur from secondary trocar insertion. These injuries are almost completely avoidable with careful technique, since the laparoscope and secondary trocars are inserted under direct vision.

After the surgical procedure has been completed, a pneumoperitoneum is reestablished. This enables the surgeon to examine the anastomosis, carefully assess the small bowel and other structures for iatrogenic injuries, and remove the secondary trocars under direct vision. Any abdominal wall hemorrhage can be identified and corrected at this time.

Principles Unique to Laparoscopic Colorectal Surgery

Four 10/12 mm trocars are necessary to perform most laparoscopic colon and rectal procedures. We do not open all four trocars until diagnostic laparoscopy is performed and we ascertain that the laparoscopic technique is feasible. This avoids unnecessary costs associated with opening the trocars but not using them.

To perform laparoscopic colorectal surgery the surgeon must have mastered the two-handed technique. Early in developing basic laparoscopic skills, the surgeon frequently relies on assistants to offer traction and countertraction. However, as experience develops, the surgeon relies on both hands to facilitate the operation. It is important to stress that the surgeon should be working through trocars that are geometrically close to each other. For example, it is awkward for the surgeon to use the suprapubic trocar to dissect and retract with the left flank trocar. Traction and countertraction should be applied by the surgeon and assistant in a concerted and fluid manner to avoid harsh, rough handling of the tissues. Laparoscopic surgery requires the gentle tissue handling techniques that are used in open surgery—especially since there is a loss of tactile perception for the surgeon.

The revolution sparked by the coming of age of laparoscopic surgery requires reevaluation of the basic precepts of perioperative management. Although until relatively recent times laparoscopic surgery was generally limited to treatment of disorders of the gallbladder and biliary tract, today's laparoscopic techniques have evolved to offer alternatives to complex conventional surgical procedures. Preliminary data demonstrate that the laparoscopic approach may be associated with reduced morbidity, shorter hospital stays, earlier return of physiologic parameters, and possibly, overall decreased cost. The myriad laparoscopic approaches to colorectal surgery mandate standardization of indications, contraindications, and perioperative management of patients undergoing laparoscopic procedures.

Indications and Contraindications

The indications for laparoscopic colorectal surgery and conventional open surgery are identical. The fact that disorders of the colon and rectum may be approached by laparoscopic techniques does not alter the preoperative indications. For example, the presence of gallstones is not an indication for laparoscopic cholecystectomy; similarly, the presence of ulcerative colitis does not imply that a laparoscopic resection is indicated. The same indications that one would consider for either chronic ulcerative colitis or Crohn's disease must be maintained. The resection of lipomas or bowel involved with severe endometriosis or treatment of benign polypoid lesions of the colon that are not amenable to colonoscopic excision can be accomplished with laparoscopic technique. Basic cancer principles must be inviolate when one is resecting polypoid lesions of the colon. It is usually necessary to perform a cancer operation even for presumed benign disease, because the true nature of the polypoid lesion can be accurately determined only by complete histopathologic staging.

We maintain that surgeons developing their experience with the laparoscopic technique should begin with benign colorectal disorders rather than with malignant disorders. We will discuss this controversy later. The common benign disorders of the colon are listed below:

- Diverticulosis
- Inflammatory bowel disease
- Infectious colitis
- Angiodysplasia
- Trauma
- Appendicitis
- Mesenteric ischemia

Symptomatic arteriovenous malformations may be approached laparoscopically if definitive treatment is not accomplished colonoscopically. Intraoperative colonoscopy in conjunction with laparoscopy can accurately locate the lesion and thereby guide the resection. The presence of full-thickness ischemic colitis can be diagnosed by laparoscope and, if the condition is present, definitively treated by laparoscopic technique. The rapid growth of colonic and anorectal physiology studies into the mainstream of diagnosis and evaluation of patients with functional disorders expands the indications for laparoscopic technique for these patients. Colonic inertia, rectal procidentia, and severe fecal incontinence have been treated successfully by resection for inertia, rectopexy and/or resection for rectal procidentia, or by creation of a stoma for correction of severe fecal incontinence, respectively.

Patient selection is as important in laparoscopic surgery as it is in open surgery. A *patient who is not a good candidate for an open procedure is not an appropriate candidate for a laparoscopic intervention.* The indications for conventional surgery must be identical for laparoscopic surgery. Laparoscopy is a tool in the armamentarium of the surgeon, but its use does not supplant the necessity for standard surgical indications to be present.

There are contraindications to the use of laparoscopic technique. Conventional laparoscopic instrumentation does not allow the procedure to be mechanically performed in morbidly obese patients; thus those patients should be excluded from consideration. Portal hypertension remains the Achilles' heel of surgeons; when present, as in open surgery, any laparoscopic procedure becomes more difficult. Bowel obstruction is a difficult problem to handle laparoscopically: intestinal distention makes handling of the bowel treacherous and increases the risk of perforation and fecal contamination. Patients who have undergone previous surgical operations and who have significant adhesions may not be appropriate candidates.

There are relative contraindications that are partially predicated on the surgeon's experience. Although originally considered an absolute contraindication, the presence of a palpable mass associated with benign disease may be approached laparoscopically. The presence of an inflammatory mass is usually secondary to adhesions of the omentum and small intestine. With increased experience, the surgeon can mobilize the omentum and small bowel. We consider a palpable mass in the presence of malignancy an absolute contraindication for use of the laparoscopic technique. The incision required to remove the specimen is usually large enough that it negates the benefit of the laparoscopic technique. The presence of a colovaginal or colovesicular fistula secondary to diverticular disease does not mandate open surgery; however, these are technically challenging even for experienced laparoscopic surgeons.

A patient with compromised hemodynamic stability secondary to sepsis or with cardiogenic or hypovolemic circulatory instability may benefit more from an open surgery expeditiously performed by an experienced surgeon. However, as the surgeon gains experience with laparoscopic techniques, it may be advantageous to use laparoscopy for selected, appropriately resuscitated patients. Several contraindications must be absolutely maintained by the surgeon early in his or her laparoscopic learning curve. Patients with coagulopathy, inability to tolerate general anesthesia, extensive intraperitoneal adhesions, and hemodynamic instability should be managed with conventional open techniques.

Intraoperative Management

The sine qua non of laparoscopic colorectal surgery is the capability to convert to an open procedure instantly. Consequently, although laparoscopic colectomy is minimally invasive, it can only be performed by surgeons with the training and experience to perform the operation by an open approach. There is no separate discipline of laparoscopic surgery—only surgeons who employ laparoscopic techniques. We will address the conduct of the operation in the next chapter; however, it is important to stress several crucial aspects of intraoperative management that differ from conventional colorectal surgery.

The anesthesiologist must monitor the end-tidal CO_2 throughout the procedure to ensure that the P_{CO_2} is maintained in the appropriate clinical range (25 to 43 mm Hg). In addition, the patient should be monitored for subcutaneous emphysema and its presence recorded. Subcutaneous emphysema is not usually a serious problem and is rarely present following most laparoscopic colon and rectal procedures.

The surgeon's loss of tactile perception is a problem associated with laparoscopic colon and rectal surgery. The presence of synchronous colonic lesions and/or other incidental findings may not be obvious on diagnostic laparoscopy, and the laparoscopic surgeon is unable to evaluate the retroperitoneum or solid organs manually. Intraoperative palpation of the parenchyma or the liver may not be adequately evaluated through the small incisions made to deliver the specimen; consequently, definitive evaluation by computed tomography (CT scan) and complete colonoscopic evaluation of the colon must be performed before surgery. The technologic advance of laparoscopic ultrasonography may help to address these intrinsic deficits of laparoscopic surgery. This recent adaptation of existing technology will enable the practitioner to evaluate questionable areas in the peritoneal cavity and determine whether structures are vessels or tubes, such as the ureter or common bile duct.

Postoperative Management

The reevaluation of postoperative patient management following gastrointestinal surgery may be the true revolutionary spark ignited by laparoscopic surgery. The classic debate of the 1970s and early 1980s regarding the routine draining of the liver bed after cholecystectomy was decided virtually overnight following the introduction of laparoscopic cholecystectomy. The new controversy, or more accurately, the persistent battle of whether to perform intraoperative cholangiography continues to be waged in some quarters. The theoretic advantages of laparoscopic surgery are that there is minimal physiologic trauma to the patient and discomfort is significantly diminished. This challenges long-held dogma regarding postoperative feeding, ambulation, and discharge criteria.

Postoperative management of patients has changed dramatically for laparoscopic and open colectomies. The postoperative regimen we use is the same for laparoscopic and open colectomies: we mobilize our patients soon after surgery, because they experience minimal discomfort. We begin clear liquids ad libitum on the day of surgery; the diet is advanced as tolerated. The rationale for this regimen is that there is minimal transient physiologic ileus of the small intestine and stomach. Consequently, if the patient is able to tolerate liquids without gastric ileus, the diet is advanced.

Moreover, traditional dogma called for waiting for proof positive of propulsive gastrointestinal activity, for example, a defined bowel movement, before the patient was discharged; with a laparoscopic procedure this is not necessary. The diet is advanced to regular foods, or the patient may be discharged while still taking clear liquids. The decision to discharge the patient is not arbitrarily established by the intake of clear liquids, and a careful examination of the patient should be carried out. If the abdomen is flat or scaphoid with no evidence of distention or obstructive bowel sounds, the patient is taking clear liquids satisfactorily, and there is no evidence of sepsis (such as leukocytosis), the patient can be discharged before resuming a regular diet or having a bowel movement.

When we discharge an elderly patient with this regimen, it is important to maintain daily contact with the patient either directly or through nursing personnel who are trained to question the patient appropriately about his or her status. Patients are instructed to return to their normal activities when they feel able. There are no contraindications to specific activities, unless so noted by the patient's primary care physician or unless such restrictions existed preoperatively.

Bibliography

Bailey RW, Zucker KA, Imbembo AL. The establishment of a laparoscopic cholecystectomy training program. Am Surg 57:231-236, 1991.

Ballem RV, Rudomanski J. Techniques of pneumoperitoneum. Surg Laparosc Endosc 3: 42-43, 1993.

Brampton WJ, Watson RJ. Arterial to end-tidal carbon dioxide tension difference during laparoscopy. Anaesthesia 45:210-214, 1990.

Corson SL, Bolognese RJ. Laparoscopy: An overview and results of a large series. J Reprod Med 9:148-157, 1972.

Cunningham AJ, Brull SJ. Laparoscopic cholecystectomy: Anesthetic implications. Anesth Analg 76:1120-1133, 1993.

Deziel DJ, Millikan KW, Economou SG, Doolas A, Ko ST, Arian MC. Complications of laparoscopic cholecystectomy: A national survey of 4,292 hospitals and an analysis of 77,604 cases. Am J Surg 165:9-14, 1993.

Duffy BL. Regurgitation during pelvic laparoscopy. Br J Anaesth 51:1089-1090, 1979.

Hanley ES. Anesthesia for laparoscopic surgery. Surg Clin North Am 72:1013-1019, 1992.

Heinonen J, Takki S, Tammisto T. Effect of Trendelenburg tilt and other procedures on the position of endotracheal tubes. Lancet 1:850-853, 1969.

Hulka JF. Textbook of Laparoscopy. Orlando: Grune & Stratton, 1985.

Imbembo AL, Zucker KA. Training for laparoscopic surgery and credentialing. In Zucker KA, Bailey RW, Reddick EJ, eds. Surgical Laparoscopy. St. Louis: Quality Medical Publishing, 1991, pp 343-350.

Kelman GR, Swapp GH, Smith I, Benzie RJ, Gordon NL. Cardiac output and arterial blood-gas tension during laparoscopy. Br J Anaesth 44:1155-1162, 1972.

Loffler FD, Pent D. Indications, contraindications, and complications of laparoscopy. Obstet Gynecol Surg 30:407-427, 1975.

Meyers WC, Branum GD, Farouk M, et al. A prospective analysis of 1518 laparoscopic cholecystectomies. N Engl J Med 324:1073-1078, 1991.

Mintz M. Risks and prophylaxis in laparoscopy: A survey of 100,000 cases. J Reprod Med 18:269-272, 1977.

Scott TR, Flowers JL, Graham SM, Zucker KA, Bailey RW. Laparoscopic cholecystectomy: A review of 12,397 cases. Surg Laparosc Endosc 2:191-198, 1992.

Smith I, Benzie RJ, Gordon NL, Kelman GR, Swapp GH. Cardiovascular effects of peritoneal insufflation of carbon dioxide for laparoscopy. Br Med J 3:410-411, 1971.

Yuzpe AA. Pneumoperitoneum needle and trocar injuries in laparoscopy. A survey on possible contributing factors and prevention. J Reprod Med 35:485-490, 1990.

3

Complications and Controversies

Timothy C. Counihan ▪ Philip F. Caushaj ▪ Joseph P. McDermott

The rapidly expanding field of laparoscopic colon surgery has incorporated advanced laparoscopic techniques with traditional surgical practice, but with this expansion of therapeutic options comes a new set of problems and complications. Complications can be divided into two broad areas: those of laparoscopy in general and those specific to laparoscopic surgery of the colon.

Complications of Laparoscopy

The complications that may occur in laparoscopic surgery vary widely, depending on the techniques employed, the skill and experience of the surgeon, the type of operation, and the patient population. This brief review is meant to familiarize surgeons operating on the colon laparoscopically with some of the more common and emergent problems.

PHYSIOLOGIC CHANGES

Cardiac arrhythmias, especially bradycardia, occur quite commonly during laparoscopy (7% to 11% of cases). This is probably related to increased vagal tone resulting from insufflation, nociception, and hypercarbia. Although the heart rate drops in many patients during even brief CO_2 insufflation, hemodynamic compromise is very rare. Many authors have considered the adverse hemodynamic effects of pneumoperitoneum (primarily decreased venous return), but ensuring adequate volume loading before insufflation will minimize these effects. Versichelen et al. considered all the major hemodynamic parameters during laparoscopy and found that while heart rate decreased, there was a compensatory increase in stroke volume that maintained cardiac output. Thus patients with adequate cardiac reserve should tolerate laparoscopy well. Patients with a poor ejection fraction, however, may not be able to tolerate laparoscopy and should be monitored hemodynamically if laparoscopy is undertaken.

Pulmonary changes that occur during and after laparoscopy include hypercarbia and atelectasis, but the changes in vital capacity, FEV_1, FRC, and PaO_2 seen commonly after laparotomy are encountered less often after laparoscopy. Hypercarbia is a very unpredictable problem and has been implicated in hemodynamic changes, bradycardia, acidosis, and vasoconstriction. Promptly administering 100% oxygen and discontinuing the pneumoperitoneum will result in resolution of the hypercarbia in all cases. Hypercarbia may also be a sign of more serious problems such as subcutaneous emphysema, pneumothorax, pneumomediastinum, and CO_2 embolus. A physical examination including palpation of the chest wall for crepitus, cardiac auscultation for a mill wheel murmur, and lung auscultation for breath sounds should be performed in any patient who develops hypercarbia to rule out these other conditions. The patient should be monitored by capnography during all laparoscopic procedures to detect this problem.

Dissection of air into the subcutaneous space, mediastinum, and thorax rarely occurs after laparoscopy. Subcutaneous emphysema occurs in 0.43% to 2% of patients. Although disconcerting, this problem is self-limiting. It may, however, be a sign of other problems, such as pneumomediastinum and pneumothorax. These conditions are also rare (occurring in less than 0.5% of cases) and can develop alone or in relation to subcutaneous emphysema. Therefore, all patients who develop subcutaneous emphysema should have a chest x-ray evaluation to rule out these conditions. If a pneumothorax is detected, treatment may be performed if the patient is symptomatic, with placement of a chest tube. If the patient is not symptomatic and is under careful observation, the physician may elect to observe and follow the patient.

Carbon dioxide embolus is a rare, potentially life-threatening condition that requires urgent attention. It usually occurs from initial insufflation of CO_2 into a vein. If a mill wheel murmur is detected by cardiac auscultation, creation of the pneumoperitoneum should be halted immediately and the patient placed in the Durant position (left lateral decubitus, head below the right atrium), and all air in the heart should be aspirated intravenously.

SURGICAL COMPLICATIONS

The use of trocars as a conduit for carrying surgical instruments into the abdomen has its attendant problems. Injuries can occur from insertion of the trocars, dissection during an operation, or during the use of electrocautery.

Penetration of a hollow viscus during trocar insertion occurs in 0.16% to 0.27% of cases. To prevent this problem the surgical team must strictly adhere to good surgical technique, including decompression of the bladder and stomach and careful induction of the pneumoperitoneum. Early detection of these injuries is critical, and the surgeon should carefully inspect the abdomen after trocar insertion and at the end of the case to detect problems. Treatment depends on the timing of detection and the organ involved.

The incidence of vascular injuries from laparoscopic procedures is 0.03% to 0.09%. The aorta and common iliac vessels are the most likely to be injured. Early detection is the key to patient survival. If the injury is recognized and treated with open repair the prognosis is good, but if diagnosis is delayed, results can be disastrous, with an overall mortality rate of 15%.

Significant bleeding from the abdominal wall and other intra-abdominal organs can also occur rarely (0.27% to 0.64%) and can usually be corrected by use of electrocautery and other techniques for restoring hemostasis. The most common location of trocar site bleeding is in the lateral lower abdomen, involving the superficial epigastric artery. Bleeding can be profuse, and laparotomy or local exploration of a trocar site should be done early to avoid shock or the need for transfusion.

Damage to the bladder and ureters has been described but is very rare. This can occur from thermal injury or trocar insertion. Strict adherence to surgical principles will prevent the majority of these problems. Treatment depends on the type of injury and the timing with which it is diagnosed.

In total, complications occur rarely in laparoscopic surgery. In three series of more than 1000 laparoscopies, total complication rates were 2% to 4%. Errors of technique and judgment related to experience may be responsible for the majority of these problems.

LATE COMPLICATIONS

As with other forms of abdominal surgery, the late complications of bowel obstruction from adhesions and herniation following laparoscopy may cause small bowel obstruction. The incidence of this problem is not known but seems to be lower than that in laparotomy.

Herniation at the trocar site does occur if defects 10 mm and larger are not closed at surgery. Kadar et al. analyzed a large group of patients after laparoscopic surgery to determine the risk of hernia by size of trocar incision and site of placement. They found a small but significant risk of herniation (0.39%) at 10 mm trocar sites that were not closed when they were not in the umbilicus. Umbilical 10 mm sites did not develop hernias; 12 mm sites were at higher risk for developing hernias when left open (8%) and occasionally developed herniation even when closed (0.22%). Clearly, all extraumbilical 10 mm and all 12 mm trocar sites should be closed. Bowel obstruction from herniation at trocar sites has been reported in several patients as well, but the exact incidence is not known.

Seeding of cancer into trocar sites has been reported rarely for ovarian, gastric, gallbladder, and colon cancer. Tumor spillage should be avoided by placing the specimen in an endobag retrieval sack or a wound-protecting sleeve before delivery from the abdomen.

Complications of Laparoscopic Colon Surgery

Surgery of the colon is very safe, and overall complication rates are low. Open colon surgery is the gold standard to which laparoscopic surgery must be compared. Currently a variety of laparoscopic procedures are being performed on the colon, including appendectomy, colectomy, and colostomy formation and reversal. Complications of these procedures are specific to each and will be addressed separately.

APPENDECTOMY

Because of the relative simplicity of laparoscopic appendectomy, surgeons have been quick to apply laparoscopic techniques to removing the appendix. First performed in 1982 by Semm, laparoscopic appendectomy was performed routinely in Europe but was not popular in the United States until general surgeons became familiar with laparoscopic cholecystectomy.

There have been a number of clinical trials comparing results in patients undergoing laparoscopic appendectomy with those of patients undergoing traditional appendectomy. Failure of the laparoscopic technique occurs in roughly 10% of cases. In general, laparoscopic appendectomy results in a shorter length of stay, longer operative time, more expensive hospital stay, and earlier return to work. Complications are equivalent in these clinical series, but these small, nonrandomized trials may not show differences in rare complications. Wound infection, however, has been shown to be lower in laparoscopic appendectomy in a number of studies. The definitive answer rests in a large, randomized trial, which may never happen in this country as more and more surgeons become comfortable with this technique.

COLECTOMY

Laparoscopic colectomy can be performed completely laparoscopically or can be laparoscopically assisted. The vast majority of surgeons perform laparoscopically assisted colectomy. Conversion of the laparoscopic technique in colectomy is important to consider: early in the surgeon's experience, 14% to 50% of laparoscopic colectomy attempts are abandoned for the open technique, although this conversion rate diminishes with increasing experience. Because of the possibility of conversion of the laparoscopic technique, all patients should be considered appropriate candidates for open colectomy and should be prepared for either technique accordingly. Complications from colon resection include wound infection, anastomotic leak, intra-abdominal abscess, bleeding, and medical complications (atelectasis, pneumonia, deep venous thrombosis, and so on). The only significant anesthesia-related complications are subcutaneous emphysema and hypercarbia.

At present there is an ongoing NIH randomized trial comparing laparoscopically assisted colectomy with traditional colectomy to assess these complications; however, the results will not be available for several years. Several clinical series have documented that this procedure is relatively safe, but it is unclear whether there is a clinically relevant difference in the incidence of ileus, length of hospital stay, and return to baseline functional status.

Concerns about adequacy of resection of malignancy, harvest of mesenteric lymph nodes, and complication rates have led the American Society of Colon and Rectal Surgeons (ASCRS) to call for a national registry for laparoscopically assisted colectomy. Until information from this registry or a large, randomized trial is available, the incidence of complications is unknown.

Certain points should be stressed, however. First, in laparoscopically assisted colectomy, the anastomosis is created under direct vision with traditional techniques. The rate of anastomotic failure, therefore, should be identical. Using the "straight" laparoscopic technique, the anastomosis is created under laparoscopic guidance within the abdomen. In the largest series of laparoscopic colectomy, 18% of circular staple lines leaked on initial test. Although the incidence of anastomotic leak in laparoscopic colectomy appears to be greater than in open colectomy, these reports are limited to the authors' early learning curve, and consequently this must be addressed by further study. Second, we can probably extrapolate the wound infection rate from appendectomy to elective colon surgery. The wound infection rate for open, nonperforated appendicitis is about 5%, which is similar to that of elective colon surgery. In the larger series of laparoscopic colectomies wound infection is not described, but should have been present in a few cases if the incidence were near 5%. In our experience the incidence is less than 2%.

It should be stressed that the reported series are of carefully selected patients, but as stated earlier, they are the authors' early cases using this technique. Certainly, as experience develops, complication rates will decrease and operative time will shorten.

Technical Tips

The complications associated with laparoscopic surgery may be categorized into surgeon specific, instrumentation specific, procedure specific, and disease specific. There are complications that are basic to laparoscopy, and we will briefly address these.

Surgeon-specific complications may result from insufficient training and mentoring before the surgeon's solo performance of laparoscopy. It is clear from studies that laparoscopic complications are associated with training. Yutzpe's review of the Canadian experience with complications associated with laparoscopy demonstrated a direct correlation to training with the laparoscopic technique in residency training programs and iatrogenic complications. The incidence of complications to the bowel, bladder, abdominal wall, and vessels associated with secondary trocar placement was significant and easily avoidable. The requirements for privileges to perform laparoscopy are undefined nationally and vary locally. The most consistent criteria are that the surgeon must have completed a course of laparoscopic training on an animal model in a laboratory and have been proctored by laparoscopically experienced surgeons.

MANAGING BLEEDING

Hemorrhage associated with laparoscopy is either secondary to direct injury of the blood vessels, as a consequence of the failure of hemostasis during the operation, or secondary to an unrecognized coagulation defect. The sine qua non of surgical management is to recognize these complications at the time of surgery and repair them laparoscopically or convert the procedure to obtain adequate exposure. Direct trocar injury to the epigastric vessels may be associated with significant postoperative hemorrhage or abdominal wall hematoma. It is prudent to remove the secondary trocars under direct laparoscopic visualization to minimize unrecognized injuries. Several techniques for directly securing the vessel laparoscopically have been described in the surgical literature. These include suture occlusion with a liver suture, direct clipping of the bleeding vessels, or extension of the trocar wound into a small incision to repair under direct vision.

Hemorrhage following laparoscopic colon and rectal surgery may result from any of several causes. The staple line from creation of an anastomosis may bleed, as may occur following an open colectomy. This rarely requires direct surgical intervention and should be handled as though the procedure had been performed by an open technique. Hemorrhage may also result postoperatively from failure to gain hemostatic control of a vessel; again, this complication should be managed as if it occurred following open surgery. Hemorrhage most often occurs during the laparoscopic colon or rectal procedure as a result of traction being placed inappropriately on the mesentery of the bowel. Babcock clamps must be placed directly on the mesentery when applying traction for two basic reasons: (1) to minimize direct contact to the colon—it is assumed that direct contact may rarely lead to an inadvertent colotomy; (2) the application of traction and countertraction closer to the focal point of the procedure allows a smaller force to produce a greater degree of tension.

When hemorrhage occurs after a rent in the mesentery resulting from traction trauma, the bleeding may be controlled directly by clips, cautery, or the application of endoloops or laparoscopic suturing.

When bleeding occurs, some fundamental principles must be followed: the camera operator must remain steady and not move unless directed by the surgeon. *The sine qua non of safe laparoscopic surgery is that the surgeon should not apply clips or suture blindly.* Significant hemorrhage may occur when there is iatrogenic injury of a named or large blood vessel or when traction causes an avulsion vascular injury. To control the bleeding, one must proceed in a manner similar to that of open surgery. The basic principle is to control the bleeding by direct application of pressure so that temporary control is obtained. Adequate exposure of the operative field is obtained, usually by irrigating and suctioning. If the surgeon is unable to gain temporary control of the bleeding or is not able to get appropriate exposure, the decision to convert the procedure to open must be made. After appropriate exposure has been obtained, there are several options for securing the vessel. For significant and/or named vessels, electrocautery is not usually sufficient; however, hemoclips, endoloops, or endoknots may be useful.

Occasionally during an episode of bleeding the lens of the laparoscope may become coated with blood. There are several options for dealing with this scenario. The laparoscope lens may be directly squirted with saline solution to clean the lens. However, when the lens is completely covered with blood so that "red-out" is total, it may be necessary to remove the scope and clean the lens externally. When replacing the laparoscope, the camera operator should reintroduce the laparoscope gradually into the trocar to gain a panoramic view and to minimize the possibility that the lens may become obscured with blood again.

The real judgment lies in knowing when to convert to an open procedure. For this reason, the basic tenet is that all laparoscopic surgery must be performed by competent and credentialed surgeons to ensure that conversion to an open approach can be done smoothly and expeditiously. We do not believe that there is anything wrong with conversion; indeed, it is our practice to discuss this possibility candidly with all our patients before the procedure. We will not perform a laparoscopic procedure of any kind when we are not given consent to convert the procedure to an open approach.

There are some situations in which it is not prudent to attempt laparoscopic control of bleeding. For example, injuries to the abdominal aorta or the iliac vessels mandate an attempt to obtain temporary hemostatic control by direct pressure while the surgeon prepares for an emergent laparotomy. Moreover, if bleeding is the result of a splenic injury and is not too brisk, this hemorrhage may be controlled by directed gentle pressure, pressure combined with application of Surgicel, electrocautery, or with an argon beam coagulator, if one is available. The criteria for splenectomy secondary to iatrogenic injury during open colectomy are appropriate in this situation as well. Although splenectomy may be performed laparoscopically for a variety of hematologic indications, we have not yet performed a splenectomy laparoscopically following an iatrogenic injury during laparoscopic colon and rectal surgery. We strongly believe that at present this is an indication to convert the procedure to an open one.

Specific Procedures and Related Bleeding Problems. There are several specific scenarios during a specific laparoscopic procedure in which significant bleeding may occur. During a laparoscopic right colectomy, we have observed that when dividing the gastrocolic ligament, or during exposure of the duodenum, if traction is applied injudiciously, an injury may occur to the transverse colon mesentery. An ounce of prevention at this juncture is more appropriate than any repair possible. In addition, when the specimen is being delivered through the incision, the ileal mesentery may be torn in the process by the use of excessive force to extracorporealize the bowel. It is helpful to determine the appropriate site through which the bowel can be delivered without the need for an inappropriate degree of traction. If there is tension, additional intracorporeal mobilization may be necessary. Occasionally extension of the incision reduces the physical force necessary to deliver the specimen.

When performing a laparoscopic sigmoid colectomy, low anterior resection, or abdominoperineal resection, the surgeon must be aware that the patient position offers a different vantage point to the vascular anatomy. With the patient in the lithotomy or Trendelenburg position with a right lateral oblique rotation, the lateral abdominal wall may be used to obtain traction when the bowel is transected intracorporeally. With this patient position the pelvic side wall appears in a new dimension through the laparoscope; consequently, the left iliac artery can be injured because of this position shift.

When performing an extended laparoscopic right colectomy or resections of the transverse colon, it is important not to confuse the middle colic artery with the superior mesenteric artery. This anatomy must be clear to the surgeon before transection of any vessel—the direct consequences of ligation of the superior mesenteric artery may be dire and life threatening.

MANAGING INJURIES OF THE URETER

The ureter may be injured during laparoscopic surgery, especially early in a surgeon's experience. The two-dimensional aspect of laparoscopy can occasionally cause the surgeon to be in a different anatomic plane than is usually encountered during open surgery. During laparoscopic sigmoid colectomy, low anterior resection, or abdominoperineal resection, the ureter must be identified. Indeed, if the surgeon encounters difficulty identifying the ureter, this is considered a relative indication to convert the procedure to open. Once the ureter is identified in the retroperitoneum, it should be mobilized and visualized through its entire course before any vascular ligation or bowel transection is carried out. The ureter must be identified when one is performing limited resections of the bowel as well, for palliation or benign disease, because the ureter may be anatomically displaced anteriorly or involved in an inflammatory process that leads to a secondary change of its position. The easiest maneuver for identifying the ureter is to observe the pulsation of the iliac artery and bluntly dissect until the ureter is identified crossing the iliac artery. If the ureter cannot be identified at this level, the dissection is carried out proximally toward the kidney. The ureter can be confused with the gonadal vessels, and the surgeon must observe peristalsis to be completely certain of accurate identification of the ureter. During laparoscopic low anterior resection or abdominoperineal resection it has become our practice to identify the right ureter as well. This has developed because of our recognition that laparoscopic dissection may be wider or more lateral than in conventional surgery. The right ureter is identified in a similar manner to the left ureter. If ureteral injury has occurred or is suspected, the operation should be converted to an open procedure.

Preoperative placement of ureteral stents is controversial. The utility of stents is limited because of the loss of tactile perception during laparoscopic surgery; however, the stents may be manipulated externally to cause internal motion of the ureter to enable ureteric identification. The true value of the ureteral stent is to identify ureteral injury. A concern regarding ureteral stents is that the presence of the stents may lead to a bowing of the ureter, which displaces the ureter anteriorly and consequently makes the ureter more vulnerable to iatrogenic injury. The use of lighted ureteral stents has been advocated, but they are of limited usefulness, since the laparoscope light must be turned off to see the stents. In addition, there are anecdotal reports of thermal injury to the ureter secondary to the light being left on inordinately long, causing thermal injury to the ureter.

Iatrogenic injury of the small intestine or colon may occur during laparoscopic surgery. The most common cause of such injury is excessive traction placed on the bowel. Other causes are unrecognized injuries during cauterization or trocar placement. The basic principle of gentle tissue handling must be observed at all times—not only by the surgeon but by the assistant. When applying traction to the colon or small intestine, it is prudent to apply the Babcock clamps directly to the mesentery rather than to the bowel. If an injury to the bowel occurs, depending on the degree of perforation, intraperitoneal contamination, and the laparoscopic skill of the surgeon, the enterotomy or colotomy may be repaired intracorporeally or by an assisted technique. If the repair must be performed extracorporeally and the segment of intestine can be adequately mobilized to reach the anterior abdominal wall, a small incision can be made with the bowel delivered externally, where it can then be repaired conventionally. Once the bowel has been repaired, the incision is closed, the pneumoperitoneum is reestablished, and the operation may be continued. Subsequently the incision used to repair the bowel injury can be used to deliver the specimen for extraction and possible anastomosis.

When considering the possible complications associated with laparoscopic colon and rectal surgery, it is wise to assume that all the complications that are associated with conventional surgery may occur, as well as new complications that are related to the laparoscopic technique. The safe surgeon should be vigilant to these complications and be prepared to convert to an open procedure when indicated.

Controversies

The laparoscopic technique of general surgery is one of the most exciting advances in the unending effort to improve surgical outcome. As with any new technique, evolutionary forces are at work in an attempt to lower morbidity and mortality as compared with the gold standard of open surgery. With the rewards of this new technology and paradigm shift in surgical philosophy, there is the danger of new pitfalls and problems. Unfortunately, some mistakes are observed only in retrospect, after the damage has occurred. This section will review some of the controversies surrounding the introduction of laparoscopic general surgery, and we will attempt to summarize the current experience with some of the more controversial aspects of these procedures.

TRAINING AND CERTIFICATION

Use of the laparoscopic technique in general surgery has become popular only within the last decade. Since a laparoscopic operation occasionally requires conversion to open laparotomy, the procedure must be performed by a surgeon trained in general surgery. The skills and knowledge base needed to use the laparoscopic technique are currently being integrated into general surgical residency programs. Recent and future graduates of accredited programs should be competent in basic laparoscopic surgery. Fellowship training in advanced laparoscopic techniques is also available.

Surgeons who have not had residency or fellowship training in laparoscopic surgery should undergo additional training, which would include didactics, hands-on experience in the animal laboratory, participation as a first assistant, and performance of the operation under proctorship.

Certification to perform laparoscopic procedures remains the responsibility of each individual hospital. A basic level of competence for each individual surgeon needs to be established by reviewing his or her training and experience in the laparoscopic technique. The introduction of new laparoscopic procedures makes the task of granting surgical privileges more difficult. Although each surgeon should receive formal training in any new laparoscopic procedure, it is more feasible to grant privileges to an individual surgeon based on his or her level of laparoscopic experience. Continuing medical education related to laparoscopic surgery should be required for periodic renewal of privileges.

LAPAROSCOPIC SURGERY IN PREGNANT PATIENTS

General recommendations advocating the use of laparoscopic surgery in pregnant patients cannot be made at this time. As with open surgery, if the laparoscopic technique is employed, it is limited to emergency situations such as acute cholecystitis or acute appendicitis.

Controversy surrounds whether the laparoscopic technique is more or less traumatic to the fetus than an open approach. Creation of a pneumoperitoneum may be done safely using the Hasson technique. The effects of maintaining a CO_2 pneumoperitoneum with pressures of 10 to 15 mm Hg and transient increases of two or three times this amount during insertion of instruments, retraction, and so on have not been well studied. These effects may vary with the trimester of pregnancy, but this also is not known at present. Length of anesthesia is a critical factor of the operation, so selecting the fastest technique is usually a major consideration.

Laparoscopic cholecystectomy and appendectomy have been safely performed in pregnant patients. Case reports of a single or a small number of successful laparoscopic procedures have been published. Not surprisingly, reports of complications have not been seen in the literature. Surgical organizations have hesitated to endorse or reject the use of laparoscopic technique in pregnancy. Further investigation is needed before a sweeping endorsement of the use of laparoscopic technique during pregnancy can be made.

LAPAROSCOPIC APPENDECTOMY

Removal of the inflamed appendix has been the standard of care since McBurney published his report in 1894. Although the first report of laparoscopic appendectomy was made in 1983, it was not until the late 1980s that this technique became popular.

Laparoscopic appendectomy has proved safe when performed by surgeons trained in laparoscopic technique. In one of the largest series to date, with over 1200 cases, Pier et al. reported an intraoperative complication rate of 0.2% and a postoperative rate of 0.8%. Infectious complications are frequently lower or equal to rates for open appendectomy. Patients report less incisional pain with the laparoscopic approach. A shorter hospital stay and quicker return to normal activities are also described in some studies, while other reports show no significant difference from open appendectomy. Costs are significantly greater than for open appendectomy, however. This expense appears to offset any savings by a decreased length of stay.

In summary, laparoscopic appendectomy is safe and effective. It may have fewer complications, less pain, and a faster recovery than open appendectomy, although some report no significant differences from open appendectomy. The procedure is relatively expensive, and it is unclear whether it is a cost-effective technique. Further analysis may reveal selection criteria for patients where laparoscopic appendectomy would be particularly beneficial.

LAPAROSCOPIC COLECTOMY FOR CANCER

After the proven success of laparoscopic cholecystectomy, surgeons quickly applied the laparoscopic technique to other common general surgical procedures. Laparoscopically assisted colectomies are significantly more challenging than laparoscopic cholecystectomy. As with any advanced laparoscopic procedure, the surgeon performing a colectomy needs to have didactic and hands-on experience with the laparoscopic technique. In addition to the technical difficulties associated with laparoscopic colectomy, there is concern regarding the proper role of laparoscopic colectomy in the treatment of cancer. The role of laparoscopic colectomy as an operation for cancer is of paramount concern for the surgeon.

Basic oncologic principles must be observed when performing the laparoscopic technique for cancer. There is controversy regarding determination of why cancer recurs through trocar site implants: Is this an unknown direct effect of laparoscopic techniques (i.e., use of CO_2, immunologic suppression) or indirect as a result of technical inadequacy of the laparoscopic technology? We have previously demonstrated that the length of resection and degree of lymphadenectomy can be identical to open colectomy. Trocar site cancer recurrence has recently emerged as a technical concern of the laparoscopic technique. There have been isolated case reports of wound and trocar site recurrence, and there has been much speculation regarding the cause of these trocar site implants. Some theorize that an unknown factor inherent in laparoscopy violates certain basic oncologic principles and thereby causes a predilection for these implants. Others speculate that such recurrences must be associated with technical factors, as yet to be determined. Iatrogenic injuries to the bowel during mobilization and devascularization may cause tumor spills. Immune deficiencies secondary to a CO_2 pneumoperitoneum have been postulated. The national registry created by the American Society of Colon and Rectal Surgeons is helping to monitor these complications. In a recently published study Whelan et al. of Columbia University speculated that there is indirect evidence in their animal model that there may be a direct immunologic benefit that is attributable to laparoscopy. Consequently, laparoscopy may be beneficial to patients with cancer.

It is imperative to identify the incidence of wound recurrence with the laparoscopic techniques presently employed. The lack of standardization in description and performance of laparoscopic procedures and techniques prevents rational analysis of data regarding trocar site implants. Indeed, the anecdotal reports of trocar site implants often do not clearly and accurately identify the stage of the patient's cancer at the time of surgery. The NIH prospective multigroup trial may help to clarify the role of laparoscopic technique in cancer. We strongly believe that in our experience we have not yet encountered a case of trocar site implantation. If this is a phenomenon that is directly attributable to laparoscopy, clearly the probability is, considering the size of our series, that we should have encountered this by now. Consequently we believe that if the surgeon has the necessary experience and is not deviating from established oncologic principles, laparoscopic technique is an acceptable method in the surgical armamentarium and may be beneficial for the cancer patient.

The Costs of Laparoscopic Surgery

As with most new technologic advances, laparoscopic equipment and instruments add to the cost of the procedure. Hardware costs, which include the laparoscope, the microchip videocamera, monitors, insufflators, irrigator, cautery equipment, and accessories can cost thousands of dollars. In addition, the costs of specialized laparoscopic instruments, staff training, and anesthesia time must be considered. The combination makes laparoscopic surgery a relatively expensive undertaking.

These cost considerations must be weighed against two important factors: (1) Does the laparoscopic technique provide direct advantages over the open technique for the patient? This is supported by reduction in length of stay, decreased incidence of complications, minimal morbidity, and earlier return to normal function. (2) Should we reevaluate how most hospitals charge the patient? At present it is impossible to accurately determine the *true costs of delivering care* at a particular institution, sorted out from the charges, contractual adjustments, and other financial considerations. Moreover, it is difficult to define the true cost of a technique that is in its infancy. Careful analysis of this technique must continue while surgeons overcome the learning curve. In the early 1960s open heart surgery was associated with high morbidity and mortality and significant costs while the technology developed to its current routine applications.

Laparoscopic cholecystectomy is a cost-effective alternative to open cholecystectomy, in part as a result of decreased length of hospital stay (LOS). Not all procedures have seen this dramatic fall in LOS. For example, traditional herniorrhaphy is usually performed as an outpatient procedure and therefore LOS is not a factor. One study showed an average increase in cost of 135% for herniorrhaphy with the laparoscopic approach. However, a more rapid return to normal activity with the laparoscopic approach is a factor that is being weighed. Reports of costs for laparoscopic appendectomy have been mixed: some studies have shown overall costs similar to those for open appendectomy, whereas other comparative analyses have described increased expense. Advanced procedures initially take longer to perform and may be more expensive as a direct result of the increased operative time associated with learning the technique. However, at this early stage in their development, laparoscopic colectomies, operations for gastroesophageal reflux or for peptic ulcer disease and other new procedures are gradually demonstrating similar operating room times, with a dramatic reduction in length of stay and morbidity. New laparoscopic instruments and possibly the implementation of three-dimensional video may continue to improve operating time and make the laparoscopic approach even more cost competitive with open techniques. As stated earlier, the costs of these new technologies must be weighed against their actual benefit to the patient.

Laparoscopic surgery is rapidly evolving as new instruments and sophisticated technology replace current equipment and these new ideas are incorporated into the surgical armamentarium. Although controversy surrounds this new technique, there are two indisputable facts: laparoscopic surgery is here to stay, and open surgery is here to stay. The real controversy is what percentage of future surgery will fall into either category.

Bibliography

Alexander RJT, Jaques BC, Mitchell KG. Laparoscopically assisted colectomy and wound recurrence. Lancet 341:249, 1993.

Aliperti G, Edmundowicz SA, Soper NJ, Ashley SW. Combined endoscopic sphincterotomy and laparoscopic cholecystectomy in patients with choledocholithiasis and cholecystolithiasis. Ann Intern Med 115:783, 1991.

Bennett TL, Estes N. Laparoscopic cholecystectomy in the second trimester of pregnancy. A case report. J Reprod Med 38:833, 1993.

Cohn I, Nance F. Intermediate or precancerous lesions and malignant lesions. In Sabiston DC, ed. Textbook of Surgery: The Biological Basis of Modern Surgical Practice, ed 12. Philadelphia: WB Saunders, 1981, p 1090.

Elerding SC. Laparoscopic cholecystectomy in pregnancy. Am J Surg 165:625, 1993.

Fitzgibbons R, Annibali R, Litke B, Filipi C, Salerno G, Cornet D. A multicentered clinical trial on laparoscopic inguinal hernia repair: Preliminary results [abst]. Surg Endosc 7:115, 1993.

Fritts LL, Orlando R. Laparoscopic appendectomy—a safety and cost analysis. Arch Surg 128:521, 1993.

Fusco MA, Palrezzi MW. Abdominal wall recurrence after laparoscopic-assisted colectomy for adenocarcinoma of the colon: Report of a case. Dis Colon Rectum 36:858, 1993.

Ger R, Mischrick A, Hurwitz, J, Romero C, Oddsen R. Management of groin hernias by laparoscopy. World J Surg 17:46, 1993.

Gill BD, Traverso LW. Continuous quality inventory: Open versus laparoscopic groin hernia repair [abst]. Surg Endosc 7:115, 1993.

Grainger DA, Soderstrom RM, Schiff SF, Glickman MG, DeCherney AH, Diamond MP. Ureteral injuries at laparoscopy: Insights into diagnosis, management, and prevention. Obstet Gynecol 75:839, 1990.

Guidelines for granting of privileges for laparoscopic (peritoneoscopic) general surgery. Society of American Gastrointestinal Endoscopic Surgeons (SAGES) Pub. No. 0014, October 1992.

Hall D, Goldstein A, Tynan E. Braunstein I. Profound hypercarbia late in the course of laparoscopic cholecystectomy: Detection by continuous capnometry. Anesthesiology 79:173, 1993.

Hanley ES. Anesthesia for laparoscopic surgery. Surg Clin North Am 72:1013, 1992.

Harris MNE, Plantevin OM, Crowther A. Cardiac arrhythmia during anesthesia for laparoscopy. Br J Anesth 6:1213, 1984.

Hart RO, Tamadon A, Fitzgibbons RJ Jr, Fleming A. Open laparoscopic cholecystectomy in pregnancy. Surg Laparosc Endosc 3:13, 1993.

Hasson HM. Open laparoscopy vs. closed laparoscopy: A comparison of complication rates. Adv Planned Parenthood 13:41, 1978.

Hunter JG, Soper NJ. Laparoscopic management of common bile duct stones. Surg Clin North Am 72:1077, 1992.

Jackson SJ, Signman HH. Laparoscopic cholecystectomy in pregnancy. J Laparoendosc Surg 3:35, 1993.

Kadar N, Reich H, Liu CY, Manko GF, Gimpelson R. Incisional hernias after major laparoscopic gynecologic procedures. Am J Obstet Gynecol 168:1493, 1993.

Kalhan SB, Reaney JA, Collins RL. Pneumomediastinum and subcutaneous emphysema during laparoscopy. Cleve Clin J Med 57:639, 1990.

Kent RB. Subcutaneous emphysema and hypercarbia following laparoscopic cholecystectomy. Arch Surg 126:1154, 1991.

Lange V, Meyer G, Schardey HM, Schildberg FW. Laparoscopic creation of a loop colostomy. J Laparoendosc Surg 1:307, 1991.

Lichtenstein H, Shore JM. Exploding the myths of hernia repair. Am J Surg 132:307, 1976.

MacFadyen BV Jr, Arregui ME, Corbitt JD Jr, et al. Complications of laparoscopic herniorrhaphy. Surg Endosc 7:155, 1993.

McAnena OJ, Austin O, Henderman WP, Gorey TF, Fitzpatrick J, O'Connell PR. Laparoscopic versus open appendicectomy. Lancet 338:693, 1991.

McBurney C. The incision made in the abdominal wall in cases of appendicitis with a description of a new method of operating. Ann Surg 20:38, 1894.

McDermott JP, Gorey TF, Caushaj PF. Laparoscopic appendectomy—review of the first decade. Surg Endosc Ultrasound Intervent Techn 1994.

McKernan JB, Laws HL. Laparoscopic repair of inguinal hernias using a totally extraperitoneal prosthetic approach. Surg Endosc 7:26, 1993.

Monson JRT, Darzi A, Carey PD, Guillou PJ. Prospective evaluation of laparoscopic-assisted colectomy in an unselected group of patients. Lancet 340:831, 1992.

Mumford SD, Bhiwandiwala PP, Chi I. Laparoscopic and minilaparotomy female steril-
isation compared in 15,167 cases. Lancet 2:1066, 1980.

O'Rourke N, Price PM, Kelly S, Sikora K. Tumour inoculation during laparoscopy.
Lancet 342:368, 1993.

Oshinsky GS, Smith AD. Laparoscopic needles and trocars: An overview of designs and
complications. J Laparoendosc Surg 2:117, 1992.

Oza KN, O'Donnell N, Fisher JB. Aortic laceration: A rare complication of laparoscopy.
J Laparoendosc Surg 2:235, 1992.

Phillips EH, Franklin M, Carroll BJ, Fallas MJ, Ramos R, Rosenthal D. Laparoscopic
colectomy. Ann Surg 216:703, 1992.

Pier A, Gotz F, Bacher C, Ibald R. Laparoscopic appendectomy. World J Surg 17:29,
1993.

Richards W, Watson D, Lynch G, Reed GW, Olsen D, Spaw A, Holcomb W, Frexes-Steed
M, Goldstein R, Sharp K. A review of the results of laparoscopic versus open appendectomy. Surg Gynecol Obstet 177:473, 1993.

Rusher AH, Fields B, Henson K. Laparoscopic cholecystectomy in pregnancy: Con-
traindicated or indicated? J Arkansas Med Soc 89:383, 1993.

Schirmer BD, Schmieg RE, Dix J, Edge SB, Hanks JB. Laparoscopic versus traditional appendectomy for suspected appendicitis. Am J Surg 165:670, 1993.

Schorr RT. Laparoscopic cholecystectomy and pregnancy. J Laparoendosc Surg 3:291,
1993.

Schreiber JH. Laparoscopic appendectomy in pregnancy. Surg Endosc 4:100, 1990.

Schroder DM, Lathrop JC, Lloyd LR, Boccaccio JE, Hawasli A. Laparoscopic appendectomy for acute appendicitis: Is there really any benefit? Am J Surg 59:541, 1993.

Scott-Conner CE, Hall TJ, Anglin BL, Muakkassa FF. Laparoscopic appendectomy: Initial experience in a teaching program. Ann Surg 215:660, 1992.

Semm K. Endoscopic appendectomy. Endoscopy 15:59, 1983.

Senagore AJ, Luchtefeld MA, MacKeigen JM, Mazier WP. Open colectomy versus laparoscopic colectomy: Are there differences? Am Surg 59:549, 1993.

Soper NJ, Brunt LM, Kerbl K. Laparoscopic general surgery. N Engl J Med 330:409, 1994.

Sosa JL, Sleeman D, McKenney MG, Dygert J, Yarish D, Martin L. A comparison of laparoscopic and traditional appendectomy. J Laparoendosc Surg 3:129, 1993.

Stoker ME, Leveillee RJ, McCann JC Jr, Maini BS. Laparoscopic common bile duct exploration. J Laparoendosc Surg 1:287, 1991.

Stocker ME, Vose J, O'Marra P, Maini BS. Laparoscopic cholecystectomy: A clinical and
financial analysis of 280 operations. Arch Surg 127:589, 1993.

Strasberg SM, Sanabria JR, Clavien PA. Complications of laparoscopic cholecystectomy.
Can J Surg 35:275, 1992.

Tate JJT, Chung SCS, Dawson J, Leong HT, Chan A, Lau WY, Li AKC. Conventional versus laparoscopic surgery for acute appendicitis. Br J Surg 80:761, 1993.

The American Society of Colon and Rectal Surgeons. Laparoscopic Colectomy Registry.
Arlington Heights, Ill.: The Society.

Versichelen L, Serreyn R, Rolly G, Vanderkerckhove, D. Physiologic changes during
anesthesia administration for gynecologic laparoscopy. J Reprod Med 29:697,
1984.

Walsh DC, Wattchow DA, Wilson TG. Subcutaneous metastases after laparoscopic resection of malignancy. Aust N Z J Surg 62:563, 1993.

Warshaw AL. Reflections on laparoscopic surgery. Surgery 114:629, 1993.

Wexner SD, Johanson OB, Nogueras JJ, Jagelman DG. Laparoscopic total abdominal
colectomy. Dis Colon Rectum 35:651, 1992.

Part Two

TECHNIQUES

4

Appendectomy

Karl A. Zucker ▪ Daniel T. Martin

Although laparoscopic cholecystectomy is generally recognized as the procedure that heralded the recent revolution in minimally invasive surgery, it was actually the appendix that first caught the attention of pioneer endoscopic gastrointestinal surgeons. As early as 1975, Dekok of the Netherlands described a technique of laparoscopically assisted appendectomy. In this procedure the appendix was mobilized under laparoscopic guidance and then eviscerated through a small right lower quadrant fascial opening for direct (extracorporeal) ligation and separation from the cecum. In 1982 Kurt Semm was the first surgeon to perform a successful case of appendectomy performed completely under laparoscopic guidance. Semm, an experienced endoscopic gynecologist, discovered an endometriomal implant at the juncture of cecum and appendix while operating on a young woman for chronic abdominal pain. Using pre-tied laparoscopic ligatures, he ligated the appendix and then removed it through one of the cannula sites. Interestingly, Semm at that time cautioned his colleagues that laparoscopic surgery was probably not advised in the setting of acute appendicitis because of the possibility of abscess formation or fecal fistula. Within a few short years, however, other German surgeons had reported the success with laparoscopic appendectomy in patients with acute inflammation. As a result, this technique has become routine in many European medical centers.

In the largest published series to date, Arnold Pier and colleagues in Tuttilingen, Germany described their experience with 624 consecutive laparoscopic appendectomy procedures. These authors convincingly demonstrated that minimally invasive surgical techniques could be successful when used not only in early appendicitis but also in complex cases with advanced inflammation or perforation and even in patients with periappendiceal abscesses. Pier and his co-workers, along with many other surgeons in Europe and North America, firmly believe that laparoscopic appendectomy offers a number of advantages over conventional open surgery. These include diminished postoperative pain, a more rapid return to normal activities, decreased incidence of wound infection, and the surgeon's ability to examine the entire abdominal cavity without the need for enlarging any abdominal incisions. The latter is a particular advantage when operating on patients with systemic signs of inflammation and peritoneal findings yet with an appendix that is found to be normal (the so-called false negative appendectomy). The laparoscopist cannot only examine the abdominal and pelvic organs but can, in most cases, deal successfully with most other disorders that mimic acute appendicitis. Recently two small prospective randomized trials from Europe have demonstrated that laparoscopic appendectomy can be performed with minimal morbidity in the same time frame as open surgery and results in a significant decrease in length of hospitalization.

General Considerations

At present there appear to be very few contraindications to attempting laparoscopic surgery in any patient with suspected appendicitis. The most common contraindication, in our opinion, would be the surgeon's inexperience with the technique. In addition, surgeons with limited exposure to laparoscopic intestinal surgery would also be advised to initially avoid the procedure in patients who have advanced inflammatory disease such as perforated appendicitis or abscess formation and patients who have previously undergone extensive lower abdominal surgery. Another dilemma is the pregnant patient with suspected acute appendicitis. Little is known regarding the risk to the fetus of a carbon dioxide pneumoperitoneum, although many surgeons have recently reported performing successful laparoscopic surgery in such women without fetal compromise.

At our institution we believe the advantages of a minimally invasive surgical procedure far outweigh any theoretic problems related to the pneumoperitoneum. It is our policy to describe in detail the risks and benefits of open and laparoscopic surgery to the patient and, with her informed consent, proceed with the method decided upon. Inability to tolerate a general anesthetic may represent another relative contraindication to laparoscopic appendectomy. Although a small number of surgeons have reported successful laparoscopic surgery using regional anesthesia, little is known regarding the pulmonary and hemodynamic effects of a pneumoperitoneum in the awake patient.

It is essential in all cases that the patient be aware of the possible need to convert from a laparoscopic procedure to an open laparotomy. It should be emphasized that such a decision does not indicate that a complication occurred but that sound clinical judgment is being exercised based on the operative findings.

Preoperative Setup and Trocar Placement

The preoperative evaluation for laparoscopic appendectomy is no different than that for conventional open surgery: a detailed history is taken and a physical examination is performed, and appropriate blood work, routine urinalysis, and plain radiographic films of the abdomen and chest should all be obtained. In our practice we also administer a broad-spectrum antibiotic intravenously just before the operative procedure.

Patients are usually placed in the supine position with both arms tucked to the side. Some surgeons prefer a modified lithotomy position when operating on younger women, because it allows for the use of a uterine probe for manipulation of the adnexa. Video monitors are placed at the foot of the bed, in direct view of the surgeon and first assistant. The patient should be securely strapped to the operating room table so as not to slide off during the subsequent position changes often used to expose the right lower quadrant and pelvis. The surgeon usually stands on the left side of the patient, with the first assistant positioned next to the surgeon (Fig. *A*). Both a nasogastric and a urinary catheter are routinely inserted. Decompression of the bladder and stomach will minimize their risk of injury and facilitate exposure of the upper and lower abdomen.

A pneumoperitoneum may be established using either the percutaneous (Veress needle) or open (Hasson) technique. We prefer the latter, since many patients with acute appendicitis will often have an accompanying ileus that may increase the risk of insufflation needle injury to the underlying viscera. A 1.5 to 2.0 cm supraumbilical incision is made that allows direct visualization of the fascia and peritoneum. Two stay sutures are placed through the fascia, which will be used later to anchor the Hasson cannula (10/12 mm in diameter) in place. The abdominal cavity is entered under direct visualization and the cannula inserted into the peritoneal cavity. The abdominal cavity is then insufflated to a maximal pressure of 14 to 15 mm Hg and the videolaparoscope inserted. The abdominal cavity is explored to determine the feasibility of continued laparoscopic surgery. We prefer an angled (30- to 45-degree) scope over a forward (0-degree) viewing laparoscope because of the greater versatility of the former devices in viewing the intra-abdominal structures. Two additional cannulas (10/12 mm in diameter) are inserted into the abdomen. *Occasionally a fourth trocar (10/12 mm) may be placed in the right mid- to upper abdomen to assist with retraction and/or dissection in more difficult cases.*

Technique
IDENTIFICATION AND MOBILIZATION OF THE APPENDIX

Atraumatic Babcock-like forceps are then inserted into the suprapubic and left lower quadrant cannulas and used to identify the appendix. Often the inflamed appendix will be readily exposed with minimal manipulation, while in other cases the entire right lower quadrant may be filled with a large inflammatory phlegmon. In the latter situation we begin by bluntly dissecting along the anterior and right lateral abdominal wall. The use of a cylindrical gauze inserted through one of the cannulas and grasped with a forceps can help break up these inflammatory adhesions; this type of gauze will also absorb any blood in the region and help prevent subsequent tissue staining, which may hinder identification of the ileocecal junction. Loops of small and large bowel are then freed from the abdominal wall until an appropriate anatomic landmark is identified. In rare circumstances it may be necessary to separate adhered loops of small intestine to expose the appendix. Occasionally the insertion of a fanlike retractor through the right abdominal cannula will help retract the bowel medially and thus facilitate this exposure.

Usually the appendix is readily identified once any inflammatory adhesions in this region are divided. If it is not readily apparent, it may then be necessary to mobilize the cecum cephalad and medially. This maneuver is often required if the appendix is in a retrocecal position. For a right-handed surgeon, the cecum is grasped with a Babcock clamp inserted through the right lower quadrant port and pulled gently toward the midline. A curved Metzenbaum scissors guided through the suprapubic cannula is then used to divide the lateral and posterior attachments of the cecum. This maneuver allows the terminal ileum and cecum to be rotated toward the patient's left, thereby exposing its posterior surface.

After the appendix is identified, it should be freed from any adhesive attachments to other loops of bowel or peritoneum so that its juncture with the cecum is readily visible. This is usually accomplished with a combination of blunt and sharp dissection. Once again, a cylindrical gauze pad may prove useful in freeing these inflammatory attachments. The tip of the appendix can then usually be grasped safely with an atraumatic forceps without fear of crushing or perforating it. In some cases it may prove useful to place a pre-tied endoscopic loop ligature around the tip of the appendix and use the tail of this suture as a retraction point (Fig. 4-8). If there is already a perforation at the tip or along the midportion of the appendix, a similar loop ligature can be used to minimize further peritoneal contamination.

LIGATION AND EXTRACTION OF THE APPENDIX

Two methods are in common use for ligating and dividing the appendix from the base of the cecum. Until recently most surgeons used multiple pre-tied endoscopic ligatures for ligating the appendix near is juncture with the cecum. A window is first made through the mesoappendix near the juncture with the cecum (Fig. *D*). One or more hemostatic clips are then used to control the appendiceal artery thereby freeing the base of the appendix. In Europe some surgeons routinely cauterize the mesoappendix with bipolar electrocautery. Although this is reportedly a safe technique most surgeons in North America have been reluctant to use this technique for fear of causing a full-thickness electrical burn to the cecum. After the base of the appendix is exposed, a series of pre-tied loop ligatures are used to ligate the cecum. Two ligatures are placed at the cecum and one on the specimen side. The appendix is then divided with scissors or electrocautery.

The recent development of laparoscopic linear stapling devices has resulted in an alternative method of ligating these structures that is rapidly becoming popular among surgeons in North America. The stapler places multiple rows of hemostatic staples and simultaneously advances a cutting blade that divides any tissue within the jaws of the device. These staple cartridges are available in lengths of 30 to 60 cm and accept multiple individual staple configurations designed for different thicknesses or tissue. When using these staples the surgeon makes a small window in the mesoappendix near the base of the cecum. The stapler is usually introduced through the suprapubic cannula and the jaws are placed around the window in the mesentery (Fig. *E*). The instrument is fired and the staple line checked for hemostasis. The stapler cartridge is replaced, placed across the base of the appendix, and then fired once again. Although endoscopic linear staplers are relatively expensive (and disposable), they are much faster than placing individual ligatures. Most surgeons feel that the savings in operating room costs (most operating rooms charge by 15-minute intervals) at least partially make up for the extra expense of the disposable staplers.

With either the ligature or stapled technique the result is an everted appendiceal stump. Most contemporary surgeons, however, were trained to invert the remnant into the wall of the cecum, and in fact Kurt Semm has described an elaborate intracorporeal suturing technique that results in an inverted appendiceal stump. Fortunately, such maneuvers appear to be unnecessary, because there have been no problems reported to date with leaving an everted appendiceal remnant. In addition, a prospective randomized trial reported in 1986 comparing everted with inverted remnants following open appendectomy found no advantage of either method over the other.

Once the appendix is severed from the cecum, the next step is extraction of the appendix from the peritoneal cavity. One of the apparent advantages of laparoscopic appendectomy is the ability to remove any infected or contaminated tissues without coming in contact with the skin or subcutaneous tissues. As a result, wound infection problems are exceeding infrequent. If the appendix is small, it can often be removed simply through one of the laparoscopic cannulas. In most cases, however, the inflamed appendix is too edematous and thickened to be removed in such a manner.

Most surgeons now employ impermeable specimen extraction bags in such cases. Innovative individuals at first used gas-sterilized condoms or the cut-off finger of a sterile glove that was then inserted into the abdomen. The appendix is placed inside the bag and extracted through one of the cannula sites, usually the suprapubic site. If necessary the fascial opening can be enlarged slightly with right-angled retractors until the appendix can be removed. Specimen extraction bags are now commercially available that are easier to use and stronger than condoms and gloves.

Following removal of the appendix, the abdomen and pelvis can be copiously irrigated with saline. Today's suction and irrigation devices are gas powered and can flood the peritoneal cavity with several liters of saline in less than 1 minute. Larger (10 mm) pool-tipped suction probes are also available that can remove most purulent debris.

Special Considerations

Early enthusiasts of minimally invasive surgery proposed that the use of laparoscopy would decrease the false negative rate for acute appendicitis. In some series this number may be as high as 20%, especially if the patient population included younger women of child-bearing age. Most contemporary laparoscopic surgeons, however, would disagree with this premise and still remove even a normal-appearing appendix in this situation for two reasons. First, in a small percentage of patients the appendix may appear grossly normal but subsequent histologic examinations reveal early or mucosal appendicitis. Second, failure to remove the appendix may result in confusion if the pain and other signs of localized right lower quadrant peritonitis return. In addition, the patient may relate a history of recurrent appendicitis even though the appendix may have been left in situ. Most surgeons have adopted a policy of removing even a normal-appearing appendix to avoid any such confusion that could potentially result in delay of appropriate treatment. The only exception to this policy would be when the cecum was extensively involved in an acute inflammatory process from another pathologic source. Removal of the appendix in such a circumstance could result in a fecal fistula or intra-abdominal abscess.

Clinical Caveats

- Early in their learning curve surgeons should avoid operating on patients with complicated appendiceal abscesses.

- Proper traction is often obtained with right upper quadrant trocar traction to the cecum or appendiceal mesentery.

- Loop ligation should be considered as a cost-effective modality to secure the appendiceal base. Bipolar cautery may be considered to secure hemostasis of the mesoappendix.

- In patients who have undergone extensive previous surgery, an alternate trocar site to lift the upper quadrant should be considered.

- Laparoscopic technique in a pregnant patient with suspected acute appendicitis should be used with caution. The potential medical risks appear minor, but experience to date is minimal.

- The controversy regarding what to do with the normal appendix at diagnostic laparoscopy is not yet resolved. However, most general surgeons favor an incidental appendectomy.

Surgical Technique

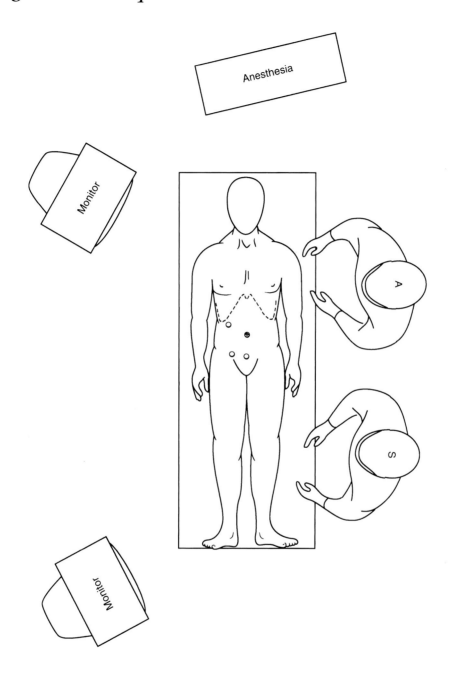

A   Operating room setup for laparoscopic appendectomy. One or two
video monitors are placed as shown. The surgeon stands on the patient's left side with the first assistant positioned next to the surgeon.
Note suggested trocar placement (all 10 or 12 mm trocars). Occasionally a fourth cannula may be placed in the right mid- or lower abdomen if additional instruments are needed.

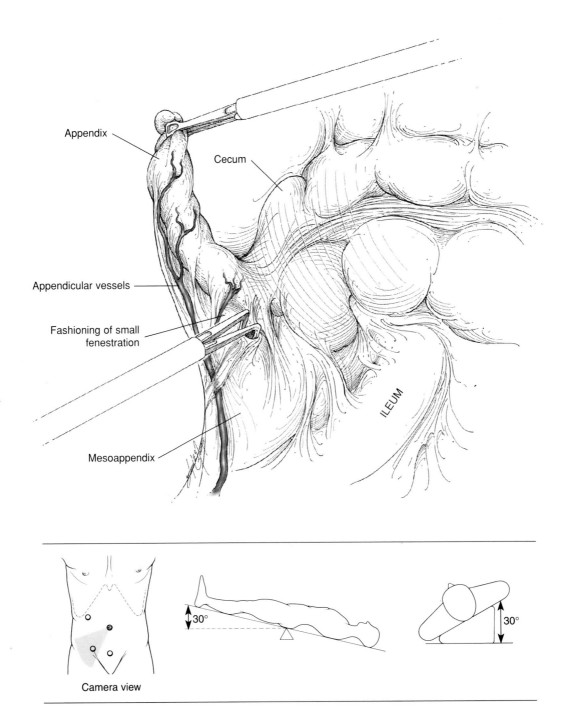

Appendix

Cecum

Appendicular vessels

Fashioning of small
fenestration

ILEUM

Mesoappendix

Camera view

30°

30°

B   After the appendix is mobilized, a window is made through the mesoappendix before the appendiceal artery is ligated.

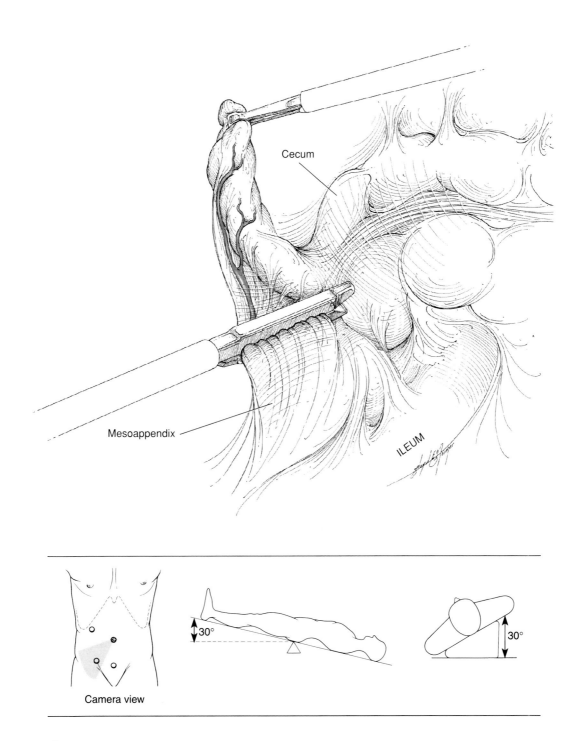

Cecum

Mesoappendix

ILEUM

Camera view

30°

30°

C An endoscopic linear stapler is introduced through the suprapubic
cannula and the jaws are placed around the base of the mesoappendix.

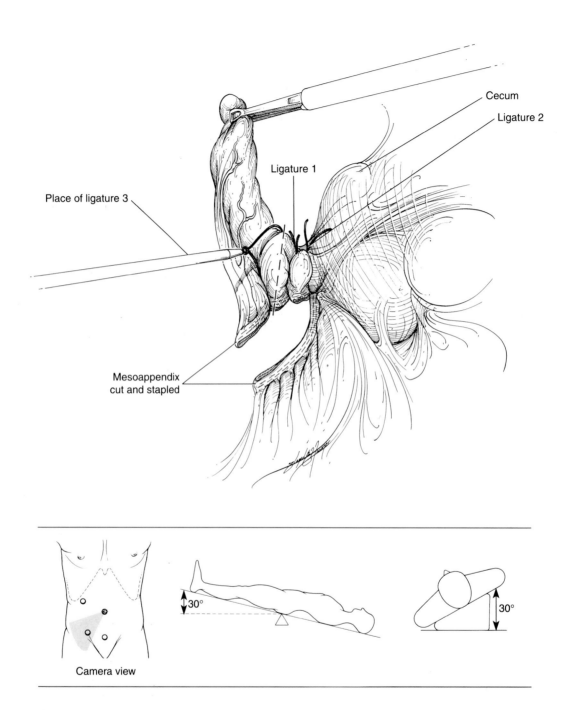

Cecum

Ligature 2

Ligature 1

Place of ligature 3

Mesoappendix
cut and stapled

Camera view

30°

30°

D   Technique for loop ligature division of the appendix. Two pre-tied ligatures are placed at the juncture of the appendix and cecum. A third
ligature is placed about 5 mm distally and the appendix is divided at
this point.

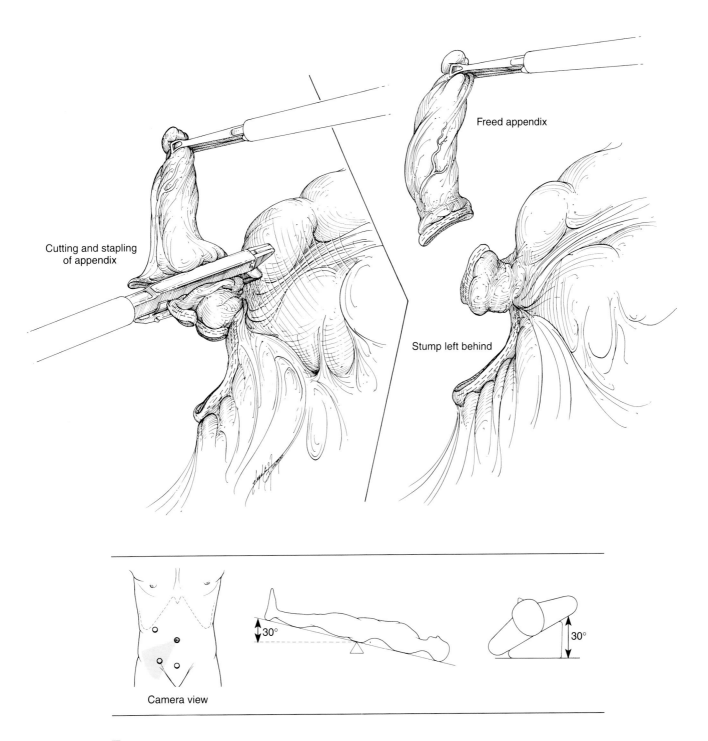

Cutting and stapling
of appendix

Freed appendix

Stump left behind

Camera view

30°

30°

E   Technique for stapler division of the appendix. After the mesoappendix is divided, the jaws of the stapler are placed around the base of the appendix and are then closed and fired.

5

Right Hemicolectomy

Manuel Viamonte ▪ Moises Jacobs ▪ Gustavo Plasencia ▪
Philip F. Caushaj

General Considerations

The reduction in physiologic trauma, immunologic response, and the cost savings manifest by reduction in length of stay and early return to work are essentially the same for all laparoscopic procedures. There are few contraindications to laparoscopic surgery for patients with colon disorders. The most common is the surgeon's inexperience with the technique. The common disorders that should be approached laparoscopically are diverticulitis, inflammatory conditions, and benign and malignant polyps. An important caveat for dealing with right colon cancer is that lesions greater than 5 cm should not be attempted laparoscopically, since the incision for removing the specimen will obviate any potential benefit of the laparoscopic approach. It is important to remember that the operation performed laparoscopically for malignancy should be the same operation as would be performed by an open approach for the same condition.

Preoperative Setup and Trocar Placement

The operating room setup and trocar placement for laparoscopic right hemicolectomy are shown in Fig. *A*. The operating room setup consists of two television monitors positioned to the patient's right—one at the patient's head and the other at the foot of the table. The surgeon and assistant stand on the left side of the patient.

Four 10/12 mm trocars are required. The first trocar is inserted into the umbilicus, and a diagnostic laparoscopy is performed. If there is no contraindication for use of the laparoscopic technique, the additional 10/12 mm trocars are opened and inserted under direct vision. The location of the secondary trocars is as follows: suprapubic (midway between the pubis and umbilicus); subxyphoid (two fingerbreadths below the costal margin and to the left of the midline); and left lateral to the left of the midclavicular line, midway between the umbilical and subxyphoid trocars. The video camera is inserted through the subxyphoid trocar. The patient is placed in Trendelenburg position with a left lateral oblique rotation (with a minimum 30-degree elevation).

Mobilization and Devascularization

The peritoneal attachments to the right colon are sharply incised by the surgeon using cautery scissors through the umbilical trocar while the assistant places anteromedial traction using a laparoscopic Babcock clamp through the left upper quadrant trocar. The assistant directs the video camera through the subxyphoid trocar, while the surgeon, using a laparoscopic Babcock clamp inserted through the suprapubic trocar, applies appropriate medial countertraction to the right colon.

Mobilization of the peritoneal attachments continues from the terminal ileum to the hepatic flexure. Takedown of the hepatic flexure is facilitated by the 30-degree angled laparoscope. The patient is repositioned in a reverse Trendelenburg position. The hepatic flexure is mobilized by placing inferior traction to the colon via Babcock clamps directed by the surgeon and first assistant, through suprapubic and left upper quadrant trocars, respectively. The hepatocolic ligament is divided to obtain hemostasis; the surgeon uses electrocautery or applies clips. Liberation of these peritoneal attachments and hepatic flexure allows the colon to be reflected anteromedially and offers exposure into the retroperitoneum. If necessary the ureter is exposed, using the right iliac artery as a landmark.

Dissection of the peritoneal attachments of the right colon progresses toward the transverse colon. The duodenum must be identified at this point (Fig. 5-1). The developmental adhesions, between the mesentery of the colon and the duodenum, are separated so that the duodenum remains in its normal anatomic position in the retroperitoneum. Next the hepatocolic ligament is transected (Fig. 5-2). Once complete mobilization of the ascending colon is accomplished, the video camera is relocated to the suprapubic trocar. The surgeon and camera operator switch positions; otherwise the dissection becomes too cumbersome. Inferior traction is directed by the surgeon and the assistant through the umbilical and left upper quadrant trocars to the transverse colon. The gastrocolic ligament, now under tension, is divided between clips applied through the subxyphoid trocar. Dissection progresses to the mid-transverse colon. The terminal ileum, cecum, ascending colon, and proximal transverse colon are completely mobilized, and the right colon should reach the anterior abdominal wall without tension.

Next the patient is repositioned in Trendelenburg position while the surgeon and assistant return to their original positions. The camera is returned to the subxyphoid trocar. The surgeon and assistant place upward traction on the mesentery through the suprapubic and left upper quadrant trocars, respectively, causing the named blood vessels (i.e., the ileocolic, right colic, and right branch of the middle colic) to become pronounced as a consequence of a tenting effect resulting from the traction and countertraction (Fig. 5-3). To reach the root of the mesentery, the surgeon should apply anterior traction directly to the mesentery rather than to the colon. If the small intestine obscures the view of the base of the mesentery, it should be retracted via an instrument inserted through the left upper quad-

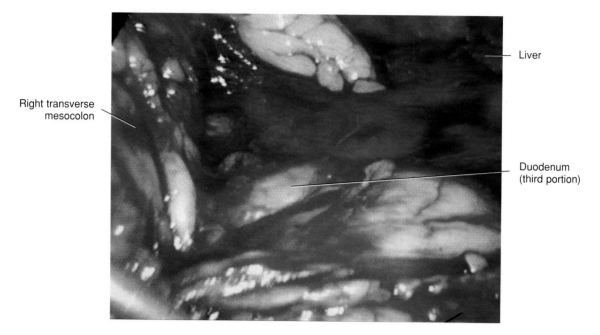

Fig. 5-1. Identification of the duodenum.

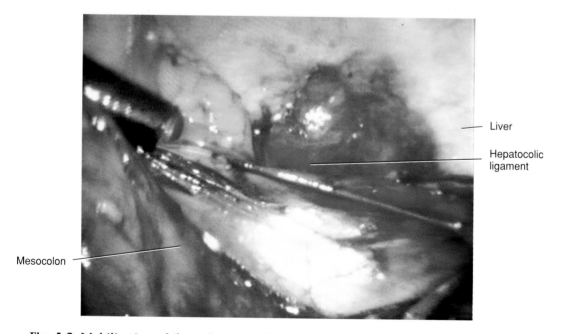

Fig. 5-2. Mobilization of the right colon, hepatic flexure, and transection of the hepatocolic ligament.

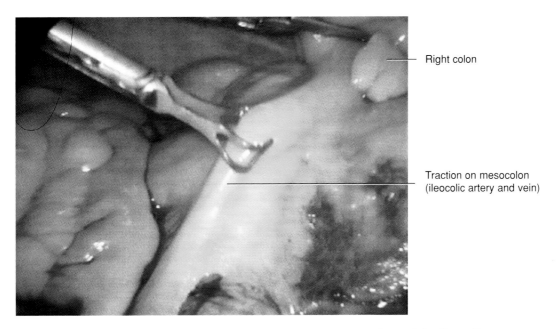

Right colon

Traction on mesocolon
(ileocolic artery and vein)

Fig. 5-3. Traction placed on the mesocolon causes a tenting effect of the ileocolic artery. The surgeon should apply traction to the mesentery rather than the bowel.

rant trocar by the assistant, or additional oblique positioning of the patient may be necessary.

The surgeon then scores the peritoneal investiture overlying the ileocolic vessels using cautery scissors applied through the umbilical trocar. While applying anterior traction to the mesentery, the surgeon, using a right-angled clamp applied through the umbilical trocar, dissects the ileocolic artery and vein separate from each other. The vessels are controlled using standard clips and then are transected. If the vessels are larger than the clips applied, they can be ligated with a vascular endolinear stapling device or pass-point ligature with a needleless Endo Knot secured extracorporeally. We do not recommend securing these vessels with Endoloops after clipping, because the application of the Endoloop may dislodge the clips.

Once the ileocolic vessels are transected, a window in the mesentery is created. The surgeon, using cautery scissors inserted through the umbilical trocar, further enlarges the window until the right colic artery and vein are visualized. The surgeon and assistant continue to apply traction with Babcock clamps through the suprapubic and left upper quadrant trocars. The duodenum is again inspected. Developmental adhesions should be separated from this vantage point to allow full separation of the duodenum and

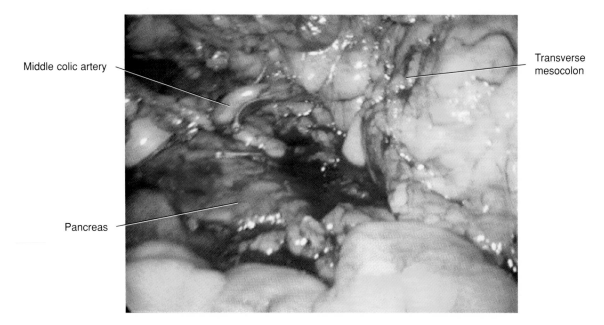

Middle colic artery

Transverse mesocolon

Pancreas

Fig. 5-4. Completed mobilization demonstrating anatomy. It is important to carefully identify the middle colic artery and not injure other vascular structures such as the superior mesentery artery.

the mesentery. The patient is repositioned to reverse Trendelenburg and the camera is relocated to the suprapubic port. The right colic vessels are then clipped and divided by the surgeon through the umbilical trocar. The dissection continues toward the distal point of resection. The next vessel encountered is the right branch of the middle colic artery. The right branch of the middle colic artery is controlled as with the previous named vessels (Fig. 5-4).

Resection and Anastomosis

After mobilization and devascularization are accomplished, the bowel should reach the anterior abdominal wall without tension. If sufficient mobilization and devascularization have been accomplished, a 4 to 6 cm muscle-splitting incision in the right lower quadrant—or, alternatively, an incision through the umbilical trocar site—is created. If the operation is performed for suspected or documented malignancy, a plastic sleeve is used to protect the incision. The colon is now delivered extracorporeally through this protected incision.

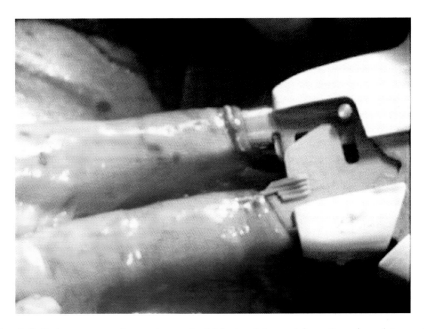

Fig. 5-5. Extracorporeal anastomosis (side-to-side and functional end-to-end).

The exteriorized colon is resected and an extracorporeal anastomosis is performed in the standard manner (Fig. 5-5). The mesenteric defect may be closed, if this can be easily accomplished. If the mesenteric defect cannot be easily closed, we leave this defect open. The incision is then closed, pneumoperitoneum is reestablished, and completion laparoscopy is performed. Completion laparoscopy allows examination of the anastomosis for torsion, enables withdrawal of secondary trocars under direct vision, and facilitates inspection of the abdominal cavity for hemostasis. The pneumoperitoneum is then released, and trocar sites and skin incisions are closed.

Clinical Caveats

- When performing laparoscopic colorectal surgery for malignancy, avoid bulky lesions.

- When dissecting the peritoneal attachments of the right colon, avoid wide dissection. The common error is to dissect far more laterally than usual; this may lead to additional hemorrhage and possible ureteric injury.

- The duodenum and its developmental adhesions must be dissected before any vascular ligation is carried out.

- The patient must be secured to the operating room table because patient slippages have occurred.

- Before making an incision, place the colon at the point of exteriorization and make the incision there. Proper location of the incision will facilitate the procedure. It is important to have the colon reach the anterior abdominal wall without tension.

- Always reintroduce the pneumoperitoneum and observe trocar sites and anastomosis before the conclusion of the procedure.

Surgical Technique

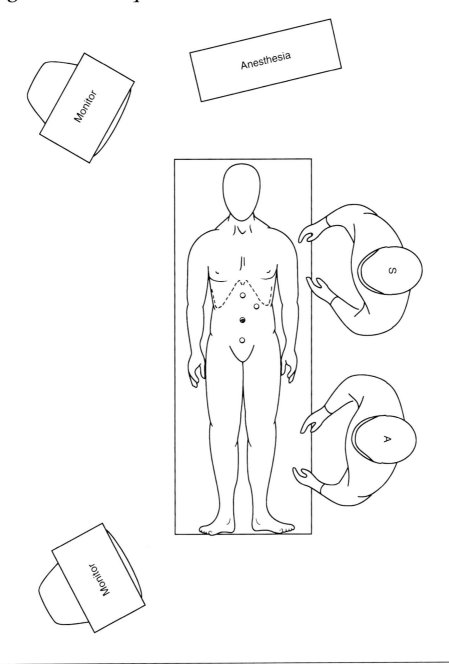

A   Operating room setup for laparoscopic right hemicolectomy. S, surgeon; A, assistant. Note suggested trocar placement.

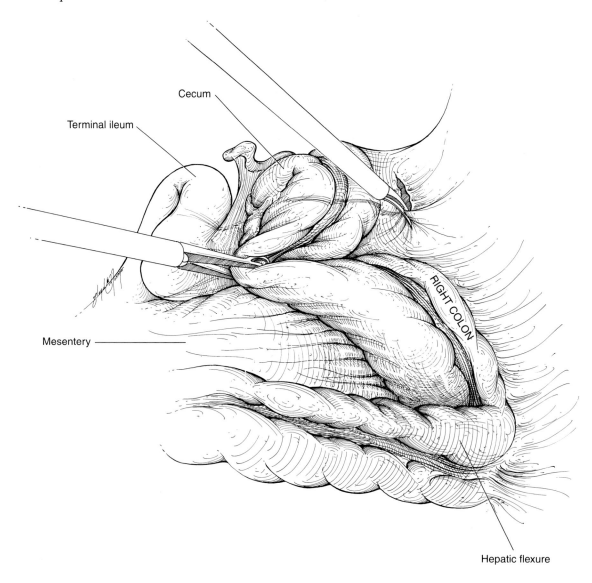

Cecum

Terminal ileum

RIGHT COLON

Mesentery

Hepatic flexure

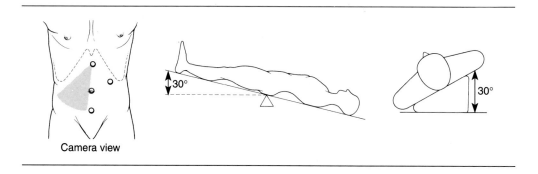

Camera view

30°

30°

B   The mobilization of the peritoneal attachments begins at the pelvic brim at the level of the terminal ileum.

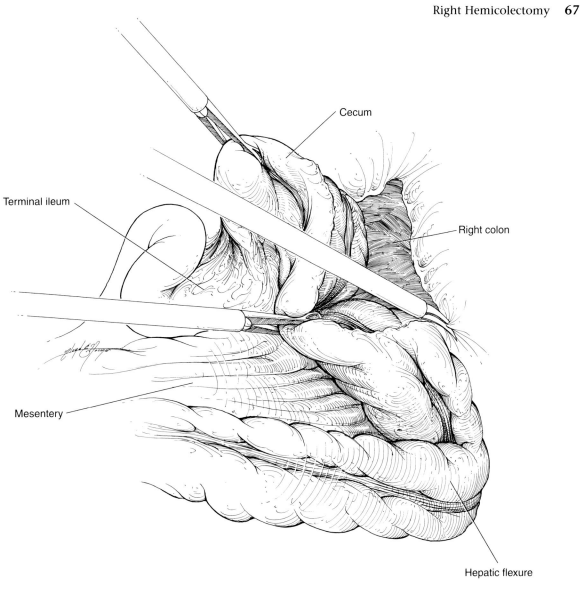

Cecum

Right colon

Terminal ileum

Mesentery

Hepatic flexure

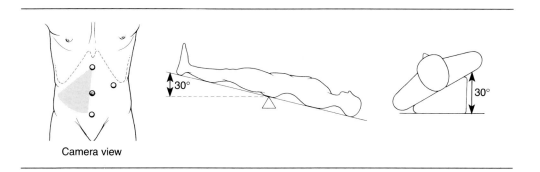

Camera view

30°

30°

C The mobilization of the peritoneal attachments continues from the terminal ileum to the hepatic flexure.

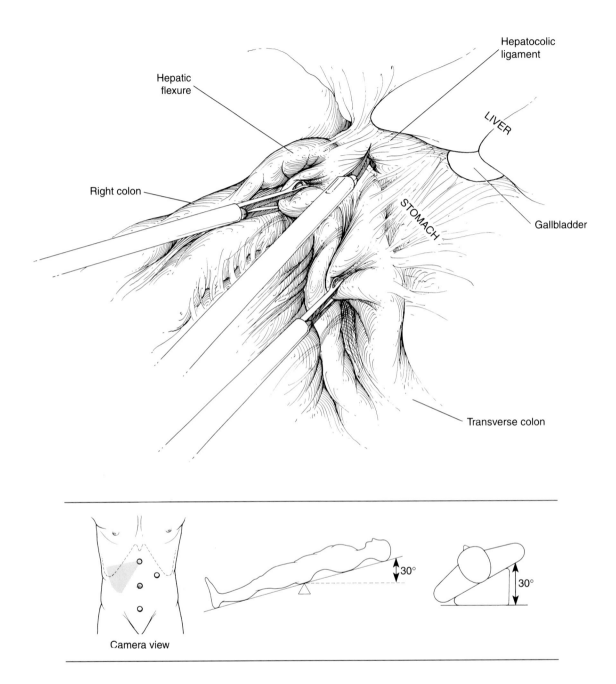

Camera view

D Takedown of the hepatic flexure. The patient is placed in reverse Trendelenburg position. Inferior traction is applied to the ascending and transverse colon. The hepatocolic ligament is divided and hemostasis is obtained by electrocautery or clips.

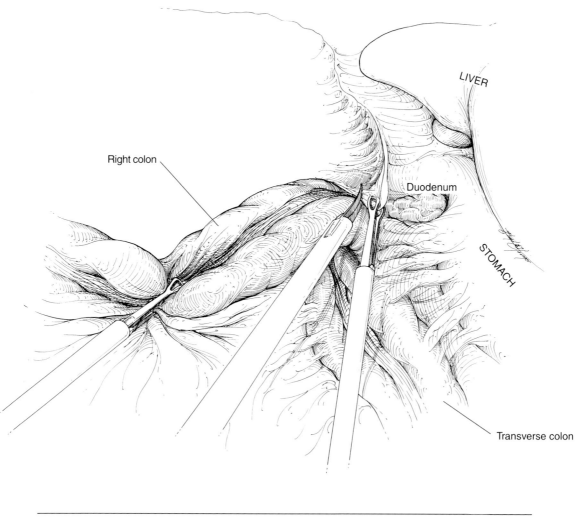

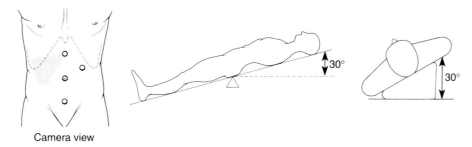

E Developmental adhesions between the mesentery of the colon and the duodenum are separated so that the duodenum remains inviolate within the retroperitoneum.

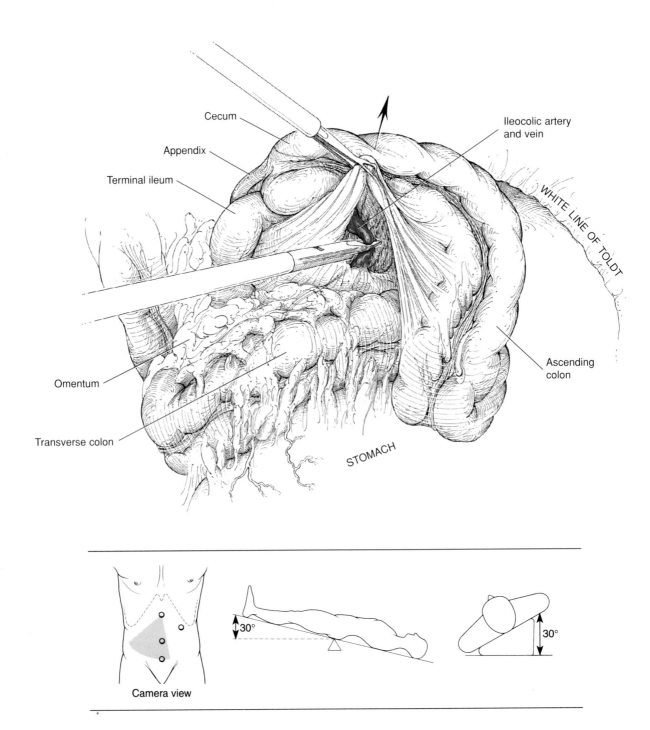

Cecum

Appendix

Terminal ileum

Ileocolic artery
and vein

WHITE LINE OF TOLDT

Ascending
colon

Omentum

Transverse colon

STOMACH

Camera view

30°

30°

F   The patient is repositioned to the Trendelenburg position; the surgeon
and assistant resume their previous positions. Anterior traction is
placed on the mesentery. The peritoneal investiture overlying the root
of the mesentery is sharply incised, exposing the ileocolic artery.

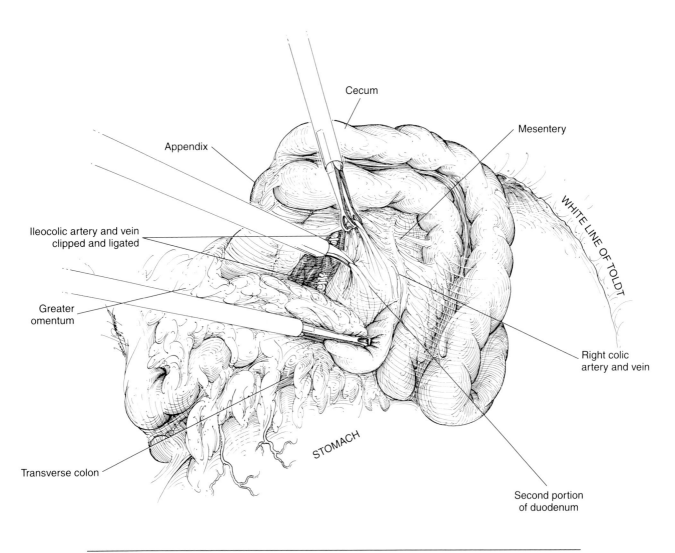

Cecum

Mesentery

Appendix

WHITE LINE OF TOLDT

Ileocolic artery and vein
clipped and ligated

Greater
omentum

Right colic
artery and vein

Transverse colon

STOMACH

Second portion
of duodenum

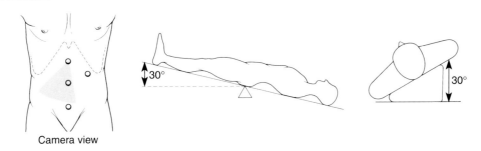

Camera view

30°

30°

G A window in the mesentery is developed after ligation of the ileocolic vessels. This allows the right colic vessels and duodenum to be visualized. Additional separation of the developmental adhesions between the duodenum and the mesentery should be taken down at this juncture.

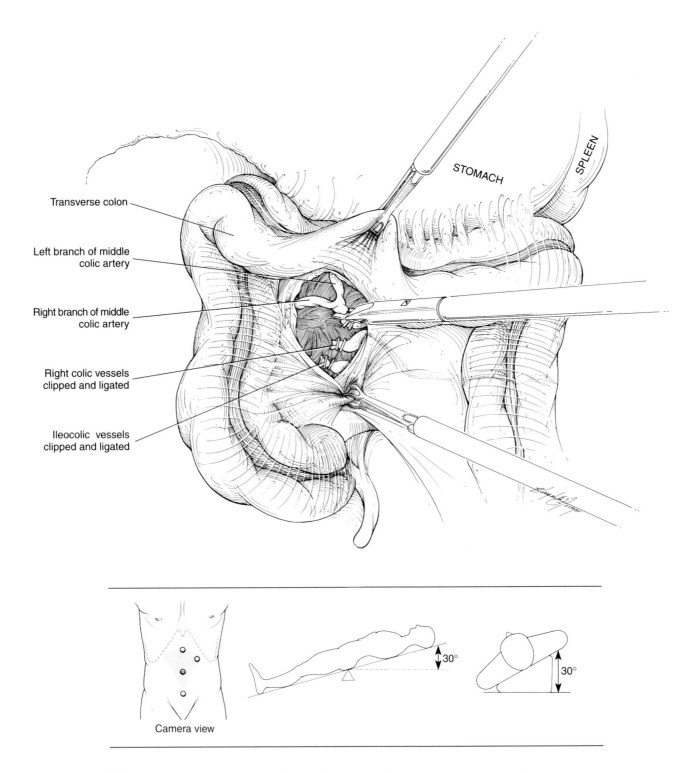

Transverse colon

Left branch of middle
colic artery

Right branch of middle
colic artery

Right colic vessels
clipped and ligated

Ileocolic vessels
clipped and ligated

STOMACH

SPLEEN

Camera view

30°

30°

H Devascularization of the right colon. The patient is repositioned to reverse Trendelenburg and the camera is relocated to the suprapubic
port. The ileocolic and right colic arteries have been ligated; the right
branch of the middle colic artery is being clipped. This completes
devascularization of the right colon and proximal transverse colon.

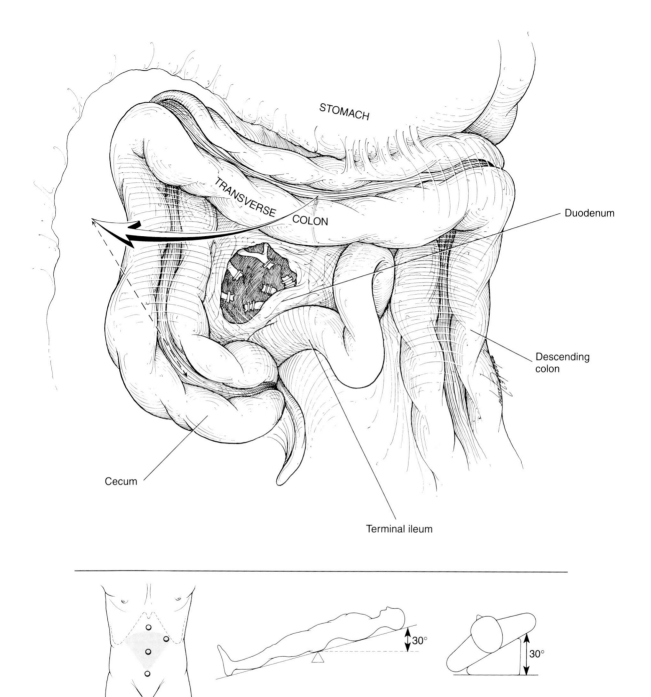

I The bowel should be mobilized sufficiently to reach the anterior abdominal wall without tension.

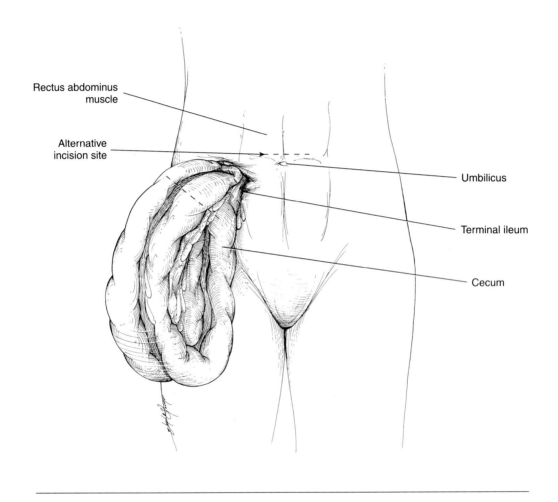

Rectus abdominus muscle

Alternative incision site

Umbilicus

Terminal ileum

Cecum

J A 4 to 6 cm muscle-splitting incision is made and the bowel is delivered extracorporeally.

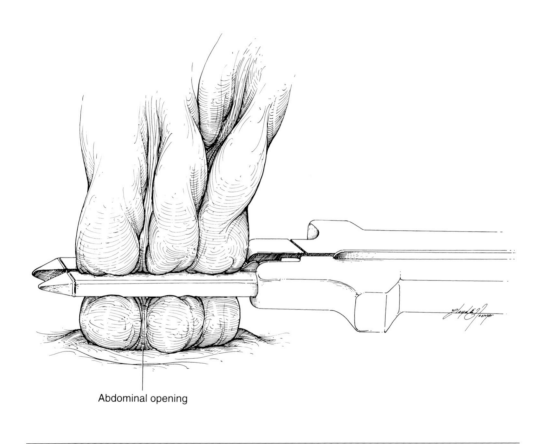

Abdominal opening

K The exteriorized colon is resected using a stapling device.

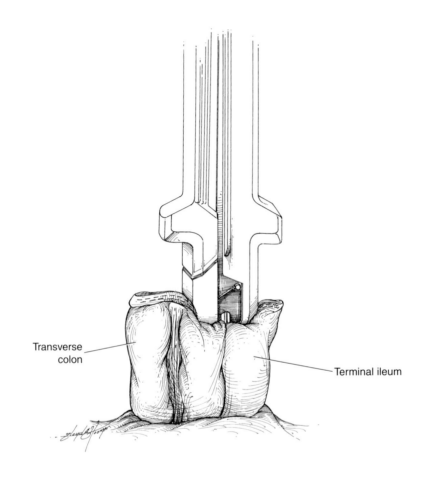

Transverse colon

Terminal ileum

L A side-to-side and functional end-to-end anastomosis is created with the stapling device.

6

Transverse Colectomy

Sergio W. Larach ▪ Gustavo Plasencia ▪ Moises Jacobs ▪
Philip F. Caushaj

General Considerations

Preoperative Setup and Trocar Placement

Mobilization and Devascularization

Resection and Anastomosis

Clinical Caveats

General Considerations

The transverse colon is amenable to laparoscopic resection; however, this maneuver is technically challenging and has limited applicability. The mobilization of the splenic flexure can occasionally be cumbersome, and intracorporeal devascularization may be tedious and treacherous, since it is difficult to determine the blood supply. The origin of the middle colic artery may be confused with the superior mesenteric artery; consequently, caution must be exercised to accurately identify the middle colic artery. It is prudent to identify, isolate, clip, and transect the right and left branches of the middle colic artery before transecting the main trunk of the middle colic artery. Ideally, two experienced laparoscopic surgeons should perform the procedure and it should not be attempted early in a surgeon's learning curve. The indications for laparoscopic transverse colectomy are few. The most appropriate is for benign endoscopically unremovable polyps.

Preoperative Setup and Trocar Placement

The operating room setup for laparoscopic transverse colectomy is shown in Fig. *A*. Two television monitors are positioned to the left and right of the patient's head. During different phases of the operation, the surgeon and team will view the procedure on different television monitors. When mobilizing the splenic flexure, the surgeon is to the right of the patient, viewing the monitor on the left, while the assistant is to the left of the patient, viewing the opposite monitor. During hepatic mobilization the surgeon's and assistant's positions are reversed.

The position of the patient is also dynamic. For mobilizing the hepatic flexure, the patient is in the left lateral oblique position in reverse Trendelenburg. The position is altered to the right lateral oblique in reverse Trendelenburg for mobilizing the splenic flexure.

Four 10/12 mm trocars are required. The first trocar is inserted at the umbilicus, and a diagnostic laparoscopy is performed before secondary trocar placement. If there are no contraindications to proceeding with the laparoscopic technique, the additional 10/12 mm trocars are opened and inserted under direct vision. The location of the secondary trocars is demonstrated in Fig. *A*. The second and third trocars are inserted symmetrically on either side of the rectus muscle, in the midclavicular line and superior (two to three fingerbreadths) to the level of the umbilicus; the fourth trocar is inserted in the left anterior axillary line, superior to the level of the second and third trocars.

Mobilization and Devascularization

Mobilization of the splenic flexure is undertaken first, since this is the most difficult maneuver (Figs. 6-1 and *B*). Consequently, if conversion to an open procedure is necessary, less time will have been spent on the laparoscopic technique. The surgeon stands to the patient's right, while the assistant is to the patient's left. While directing the video camera through the left midclavicular trocar, the assistant applies traction downward and medially with a Babcock clamp in the left axillary line trocar, to the descending colon and splenic flexure. The surgeon retracts the splenic flexure superiorly and medially using a Babcock clamp inserted through the right midclavicular trocar. Traction is directed to deliver the descending colon and splenic flexure to the midline. With cautery scissors placed in the umbilical trocar, the surgeon incises the peritoneal attachments of the left colon and proceeds proximally toward the splenic flexure, dividing the splenocolic and renocolic ligaments with cautery scissors. Occasionally these ligaments will need to be divided between clips, with the clip applier inserted through the umbilical trocar. A spatula or right-angle clamp is used to gently push the descending colon medially and the splenic flexure caudally. Dissection proceeds toward the gastrocolic ligament, with downward traction provided by the assistant to the transverse colon. Countertraction is applied by the surgeon to the superior edge of the gastrocolic ligament until the gastroepiploic vessels are identified and divided between clips.

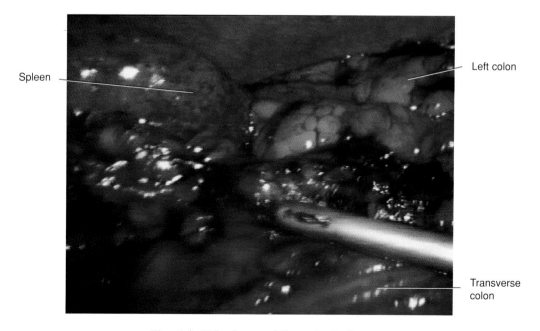

Fig. 6-1. Takedown of the splenic flexure.

Once the distal transverse colon is adequately mobilized and takedown of the splenic flexure is accomplished, the surgeon and assistant change positions. The assistant now directs the video camera through the umbilical trocar while applying caudal and inferior traction to the ascending colon through the right midclavicular trocar. The surgeon places a Babcock clamp through the left midclavicular trocar for inferior countertraction to the proximal transverse colon. The peritoneal attachments of the ascending colon are incised with cautery scissors, placed through the left anterior axillary trocar, and dissection proceeds toward the hepatic flexure. The hepatocolic ligament is transected using the cautery scissors, which remain in the left axillary trocar, although if necessary, the scissors can be exchanged for a clip applier. The right transverse colon is mobilized by continuing the downward traction from a Babcock clamp directed by the surgeon through the left midclavicular trocar, while the assistant offers countertraction to the superior edge of the gastrocolic ligament or the inferior border of the stomach with a Babcock clamp placed through the right midclavicular trocar. Most of this dissection can be accomplished using cautery scissors; however, larger vessels must be clipped before transection. The mobilization of the ascending colon and hepatic flexure completed, the transverse colon is now fully mobilized. The duodenum is now identified by separating the developmental adhesions and developing the natural plane that exists between the duodenum and mesentery. This dissection will serve as a guide to the root of the middle colic vessels.

At this point the surgeon will decide whether the greater omentum should be removed. If the greater omentum is not to be removed, the greater omentum is separated from the transverse colon by applying superior traction to the greater omentum while inferior countertraction to the transverse colon is applied by the surgeon and assistant. The dissection in the avascular plane between the transverse colon and the greater omentum is not very time-consuming and is performed using cautery scissors.

Devascularization is the most treacherous aspect of this procedure. Anterior traction is placed on the mesentery with Babcock clamps applied through the right midclavicular trocar and the left axillary trocar, by the surgeon and assistant, respectively. This will cause the middle colic vessels to bow like violin strings. The mesentery may be thicker in the distribution of the middle colic artery and, even with traction, the artery may be difficult to identify. Transillumination of the mesentery is not useful; however, an ultrasound probe may be helpful in identifying the middle colic artery. Accurate identification of the middle colic vessels is important, since the superior mesenteric vessels can be confused for the middle colic vessels. The superior mesenteric vessels can be adherent or near the middle colic vessels, and as dissection in this area may lead to a direction farther superior and dorsal than the surgeon intends, and the superior mesenteric vessels can be mistakenly divided. This is a disastrous complication.

The mesentery of the transverse colon is scored and the artery and vein are individually isolated with a right angle clamp inserted through the umbilical trocar, while the surgeon provides traction to the mesentery via a Babcock clamp placed through the right midclavicular trocar. The assistant directs the video camera through the left midclavicular trocar and provides anterior traction with a Babcock clamp placed in the left anterior axillary trocar. Once isolated, the middle colic vessels are clipped individually at the base of the vessels using several clips on the mesenteric side and one clip on the specimen side of each vessel. If the middle colic artery is too large for the clips to completely occlude it, other options for hemostasis should be considered. An endolinear vascular stapling device may be used to control the vessel, or an intracorporeal or extracorporeal suturing technique may be employed.

Resection and Anastomosis

After mobilization and devascularization of the bowel is accomplished, the bowel is directed to the anterior abdominal wall to ascertain the adequacy of mobilization. If it is adequate, a 4 to 5 cm transverse incision is made in the epigastrium. An alternative incision can also be used. The rectus muscles are separated from either side of the midline, and the abdomen is entered through either a transverse or midline incision of the fascia and peritoneum. The transverse colon is delivered through the incision, resected in a standard manner, and a stapled, side-to-side anastomosis created. A handsewn technique may also be used if cost is a consideration. The completed anastomosis is returned to the abdominal cavity. We make no attempt to close the mesenteric defect. The incision is closed and the pneumoperitoneum is reestablished. The anastomosis is examined for possible torsion and hemostasis is obtained. The secondary trocars are removed under direct vision. The operation is completed with closure of all incisions.

Clinical Caveats

- Mobilization of the splenic flexure should be undertaken as the first part of this procedure. This is the most difficult maneuver; thus, by performing it first, if conversion to an open procedure is required, this will be evident early in the procedure.

- The clinical decision whether to remove the greater omentum is important and should be based on the clinical indications for the procedure preoperatively.

- Devascularization is the most treacherous aspect of this procedure. Accurate identification of the middle colic vessels is important since the superior mesenteric vessels can be mistakenly identified and ligated, with disastrous outcome.

Surgical Technique

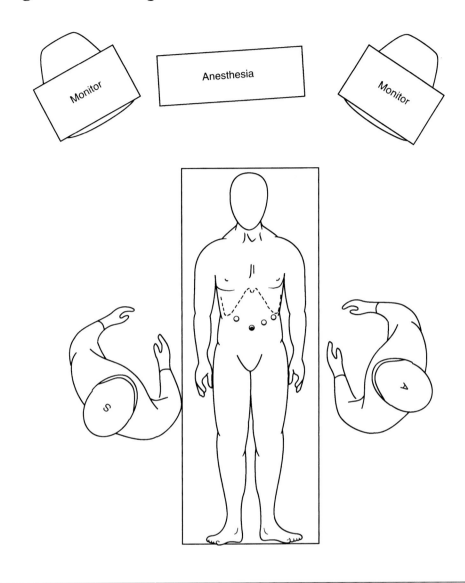

A   Operating room setup for laparoscopic transverse colectomy. Note suggested trocar placement for transverse colectomy.

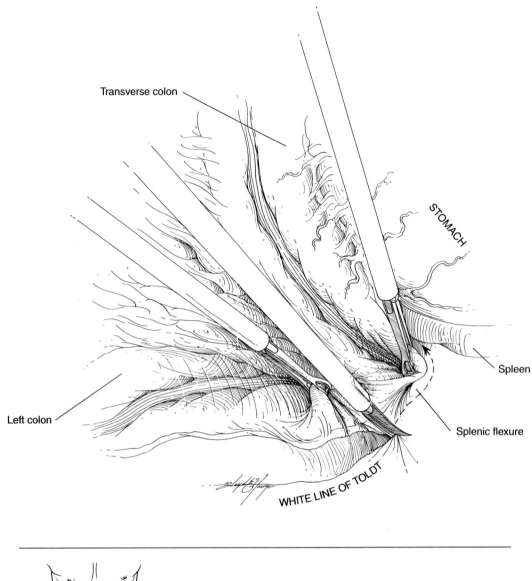

Transverse colon

STOMACH

Spleen

Splenic flexure

Left colon

WHITE LINE OF TOLDT

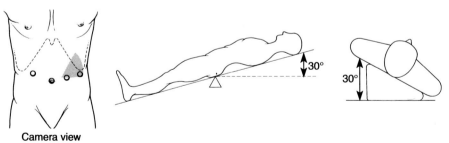

30°

30°

Camera view

B Mobilization of the splenic flexure. Traction is applied to deliver the
descending colon and splenic flexure to the midline. Cautery scissors
are used to incise the peritoneal attachments—to splenocolic and
phrenocolic ligaments.

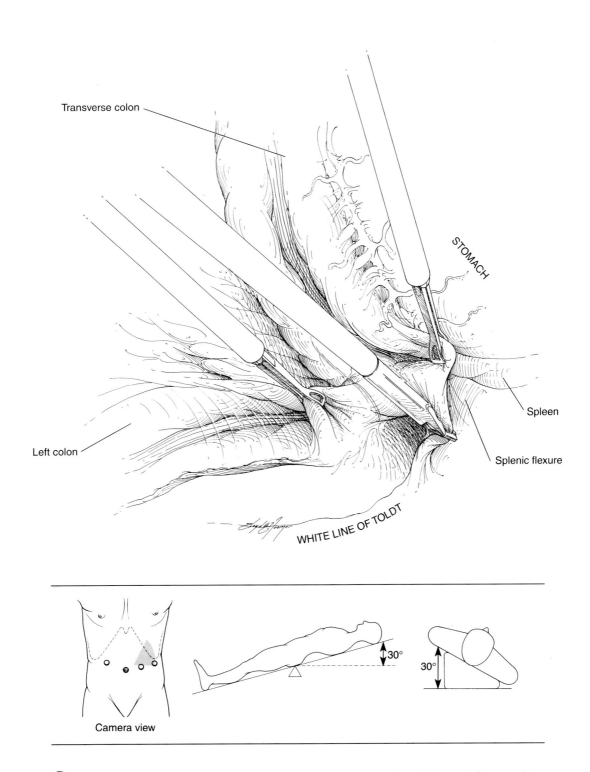

Transverse colon

STOMACH

Spleen

Splenic flexure

Left colon

WHITE LINE OF TOLDT

Camera view

30°

30°

C The splenocolic and phrenocolic ligaments are divided with hemoclips or cautery scissors.

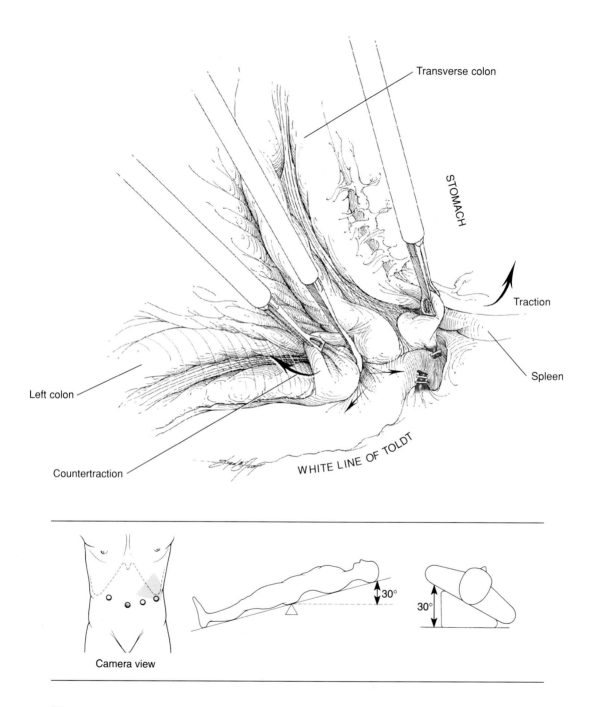

Transverse colon

STOMACH

Traction

Spleen

Left colon

Countertraction

WHITE LINE OF TOLDT

Camera view

30°

30°

D   Traction is applied to the superior edge of the gastrocolic ligament while countertraction is applied to the distal transverse colon and splenic flexure inferiorly.

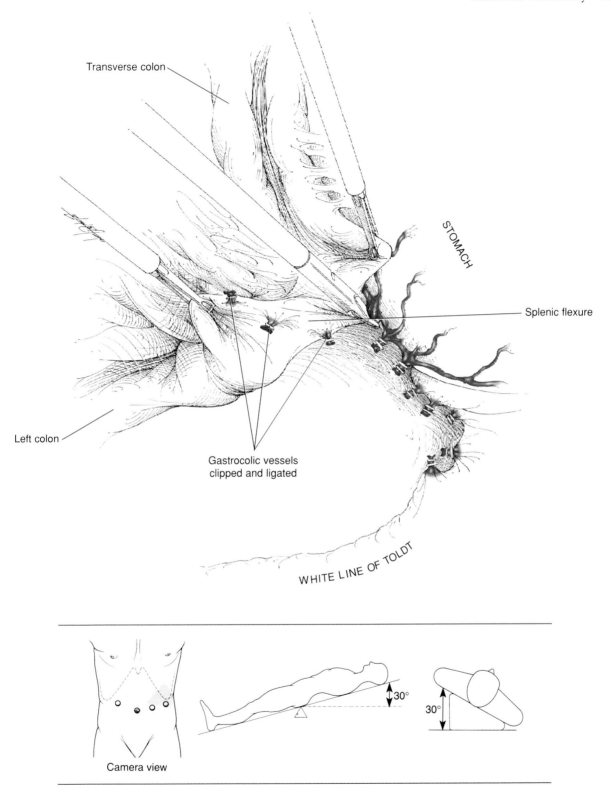

Transverse colon

STOMACH

Splenic flexure

Left colon

Gastrocolic vessels
clipped and ligated

WHITE LINE OF TOLDT

Camera view

30°

30°

E   Ligation of the gastrocolic ligament.

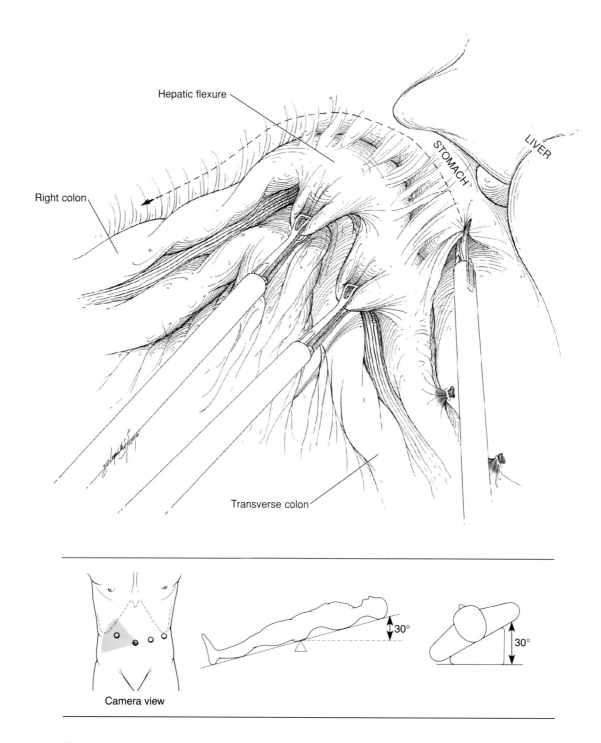

Hepatic flexure

Right colon

LIVER

STOMACH

Transverse colon

Camera view

30°

30°

F Takedown of the hepatic flexure.

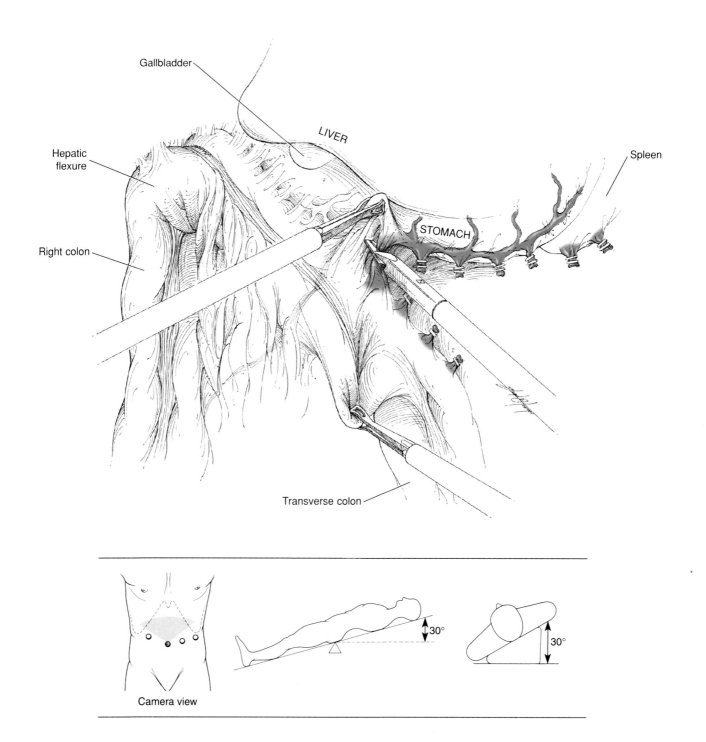

G   The proximal gastrocolic ligament is divided to complete the take-down of the hepatic flexure.

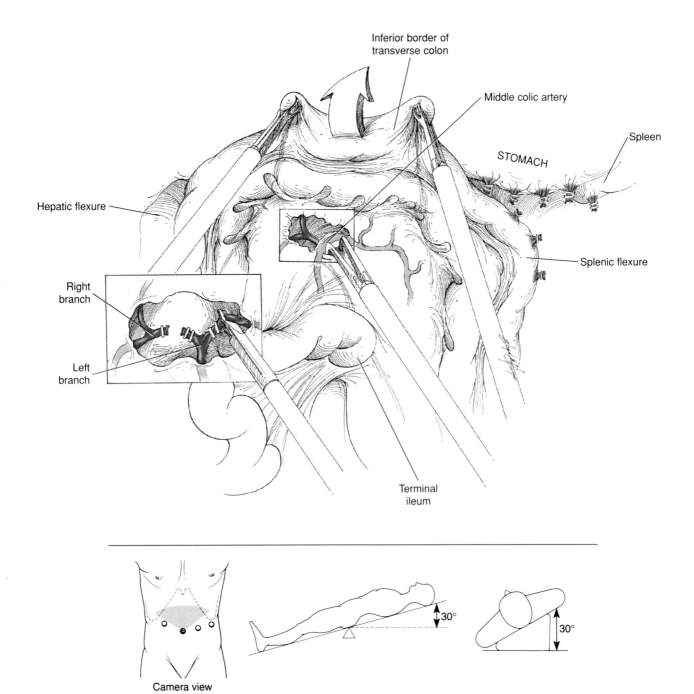

H Devascularization of the middle colic artery. Anterior traction is placed on the mesentery, and the peritoneal lining of the mesentery is scored. A right-angle clamp is used to dissect the right and left branches of the middle colic vessels. These branches are clipped and divided.

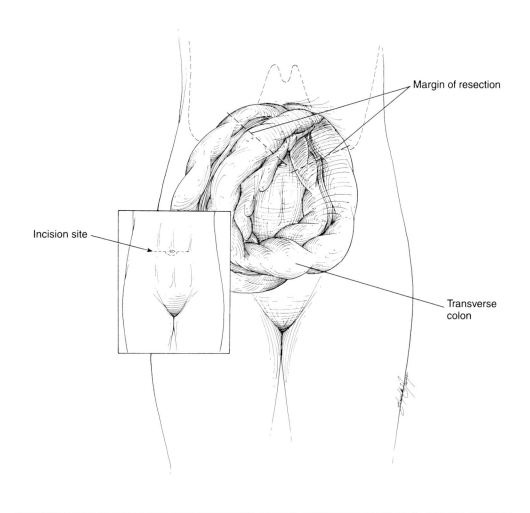

Margin of resection

Incision site

Transverse colon

I   A 4 to 5 cm incision is made in the epigastrium. This is a muscle-splitting incision with retraction of the rectus. The transverse colon is exteriorized through this incision. *Inset:* Incision site.

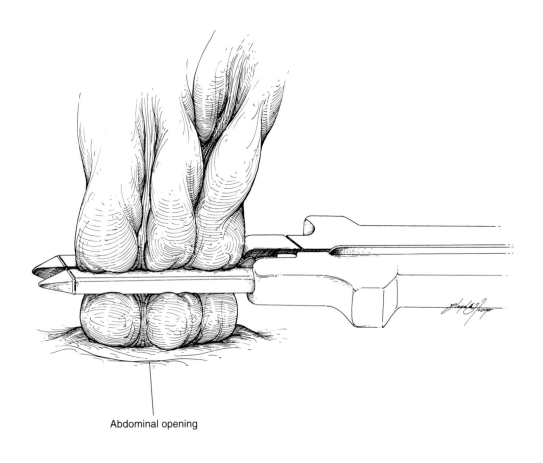

Abdominal opening

J   The bowel and mesentery are transected with a stapling device. The specimen is removed from the field.

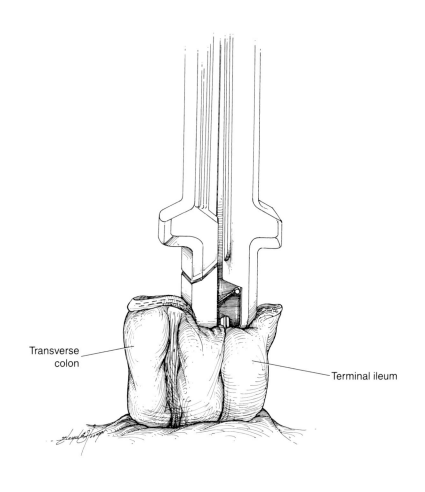

K Side-to-side and functional end-to-end anastomosis created with the stapling device.

7

Left Hemicolectomy

Rene F. Hartmann ▪ Philip F. Caushaj ▪ Moises Jacobs ▪
Gustavo Plasencia

General Considerations

Preoperative Setup and Trocar Placement

Mobilization and Devascularization

Resection and Anastomosis

Resection of the Left and Sigmoid Colon

Clinical Caveats

General Considerations

The takedown of the splenic flexure of the colon is the most technically demanding aspect of this procedure. The inexperienced surgeon should employ considerable caution dividing the splenocolic and phrenocolic ligaments. It is often necessary to change the vantage point to view this portion of the procedure. The ureter should be identified as an integral part of this procedure. The indications and contraindications are the same; however, the caveat should be to avoid bulky lesions.

Preoperative Setup and Trocar Placement

The operating room setup for laparoscopic left colectomy and takedown of the splenic flexure is demonstrated in Fig. *A*. Two television monitors are positioned to the left of the patient—one at the head and the other at the feet. The surgeon stands to the patient's right, while the assistant stands to the left or between the legs. The patient is placed in the modified lithotomy position and secured to the operating room table. The table is placed in the Trendelenburg and left lateral oblique position.

A CO_2 pneumoperitoneum is established by standard methods. The trocars that will be required initially are 10/12 mm in size. The first trocar is placed infraumbilically and the laparoscope is inserted. A diagnostic laparoscopy is performed. If there is no contraindication to proceeding with the laparoscopic technique, the additional 10/12 mm trocars are opened and inserted under direct vision. The secondary trocars are placed (Fig. *A*): at the epigastrium; suprapubically off the midline to the left; and in the left flank at the level of the umbilicus.

Mobilization and Devascularization

Once all trocars are in place, the video camera is relocated to the epigastric trocar; at the same time, the assistant inserts a Babcock clamp through the left flank trocar, which will supply traction to the descending colon. The surgeon inserts a Babcock clamp through the umbilical trocar and cautery scissors through the suprapubic trocar.

Mobilization of the colon begins by incising the peritoneal attachments of the midsigmoid colon and proceeds proximally toward the splenic flexure. Both surgeon and assistant view the monitor at the patient's feet. The colon is retracted medially and the left ureter identified.

When the peritoneal attachments have been incised to the level of the splenic flexure, the position of the operating room table is changed to a reverse Trendelenburg position with left lateral oblique rotation. The 0-degree laparoscope is removed and a 30-degree angled laparoscope is inserted through the suprapubic trocar. The assistant then moves between the patient's legs, directs the video camera, and provides lateral countertraction to the bowel at the splenocolic and phrenocolic ligaments with a Babcock clamp through the left flank trocar. The surgeon retracts the splenic flexure medially with a Babcock clamp inserted through the epigastric trocar, placing the phrenocolic and splenocolic ligaments under tension. These ligaments are transected, with cautery scissors or between clips, through the umbilical trocar. During this portion of the procedure, the surgeon and assistant view the monitor at the patient's head.

After these ligaments are transected, the OR team and patient remain in the same positions. The assistant will provide traction to the inferior edge of the gastrocolic ligament with a Babcock clamp inserted through the left flank trocar. The surgeon transects the gastrocolic ligament to the level of the midtransverse colon with cautery scissors and a clip applier inserted through the umbilical trocar. This dissection continues to the splenic flexure. If there is no clinical indication for resection of the greater omentum, the technical approach changes: the assistant will apply traction to the transverse colon inferiorly with a Babcock clamp inserted through the left flank trocar while the surgeon applies countertraction to the greater omentum superiorly with a Babcock clamp inserted through the epigastric trocar. This allows separation of the greater omentum from the transverse colon with cautery scissors applied by the surgeon through the umbilical trocar.

When the left colon is completely mobilized (Figs. 7-1 through 7-3) and the splenic flexure liberated from its attachments, the bowel is delivered to the anterior abdominal wall to determine whether mobilization is adequate to deliver the colon through an incision. A muscle-splitting incision of 4 to 5 cm is made in the left flank, incorporating the left flank trocar site. Extracorporeal devascularization, bowel resection, and anastomosis are performed through this incision. The contents of the peritoneal cavity are explored manually at this juncture, if possible.

Intracorporeal devascularization is indicated to enable complete mobilization and delivery of the bowel through the incision or to follow basic oncologic principles. Thus, when intracorporeal devascularization is needed, the mobilized colon is reflected laterally before the muscle-splitting incision is made.

Until this point the goal has been to make the left colon a midline structure. The assistant directs the video camera through the suprapubic

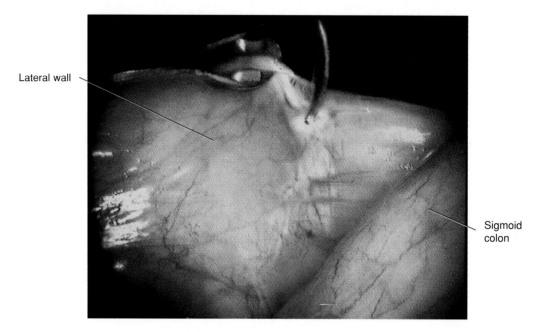

Lateral wall

Sigmoid colon

Fig. 7-1. Lateral mobilization of the left colon.

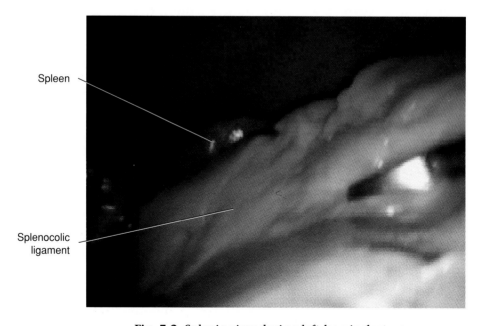

Spleen

Splenocolic ligament

Fig. 7-2. Splenic view during left hemicolectomy.

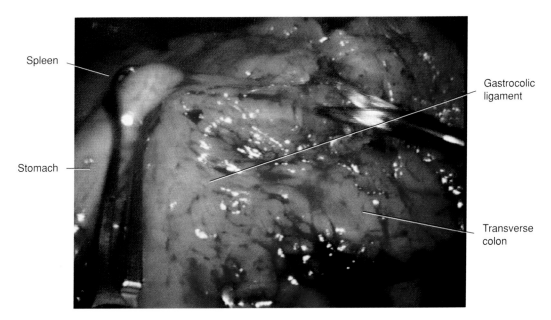

Spleen

Stomach

Gastrocolic
ligament

Transverse
colon

Fig. 7-3. Takedown of the gastrocolic ligament.

trocar while placing the mesentery of the colon under traction with a Babcock clamp inserted through the left flank trocar. The surgeon applies countertraction to the mesentery by a Babcock clamp through the epigastric trocar, then scores the peritoneal lining of the mesentery at the anatomic level of the left colic artery or the inferior mesenteric artery with cautery scissors placed through the umbilical trocar. The traction and countertraction applied to the mesentery will cause the vessels to bow like violin strings, thus directing the surgeon. The dissection is continued with cautery scissors proximally along the base of the mesentery to the mid-transverse colon through the umbilical trocar. The left colic or inferior mesenteric vessels are divided between clips, applied through the umbilical trocar, thereby creating a mesenteric window at the base of the mesentery.

Caution must be exercised before vascular ligation to reidentify the left ureter. The perspective of devascularization becomes clearer once this window is created. The surgeon continues the devascularization proximally to the left branch of the middle colic artery. The anatomic location of the middle colic vessels must be clear to the surgeon. If there is any question regarding the anatomic location of the middle colic vessels, this must be resolved before continuing devascularization. Iatrogenic injury to the superior mesenteric vessels is also possible. Once the left branch of the middle colic vessels are divided between clips, the small vascular branches and the marginal artery are also divided until the colon is devascularized and cleared of fat and mesentery at the proximal margin of resection. This completes the intracorporeal devascularization.

Resection and Anastomosis

After mobilization (and intracorporeal devascularization, if necessary), a 4 to 5 cm muscle-splitting incision is made in the left flank incorporating the left flank trocar site. The colon is delivered through this incision and a functional end-to-end anastomosis is fashioned. The bowel is returned to the peritoneal cavity and the incision is closed. The pneumoperitoneum is reestablished and the anastomosis is examined. After ensuring that hemostasis is adequate and that no torsion of the bowel exists, the secondary trocars are removed under direct vision.

Resection of the Left and Sigmoid Colon

If the procedure is a formal left hemicolectomy and includes the removal of the sigmoid colon, the procedure proceeds as described. However, the peritoneal attachments of the sigmoid colon are completely incised. The suprapubic 10/12 mm trocar is exchanged for a 33 mm trocar and an endolinear cutter is used, with separate firings, to divide the mesorectum and colon at the rectosigmoid junction. This extension of the operation proceeds as described in Chapter 8.

Clinical Caveats

- The patient must be placed in the lithotomy position for this procedure to be performed completely.

- It is necessary to change the surgeon's viewing perspective, with the television monitor placed at the head of the table. As the surgeon gains experience with the procedure, the anatomic view of the splenic flexure is ideal, and parenthetically, superior to that of open procedures.

- The separation of the greater omentum from the distal transverse colon is easily accomplished by placing traction on the greater omentum and countertraction to the mesentery of the transverse colon.

- The left ureter must be identified before any vascular ligation to minimize the potential for iatrogenic injuries.

- Intraoperative colonoscopy may be necessary to ascertain the location of the lesion as well as the margins of resection. The operating room should be set up for this possibility.

Surgical Technique

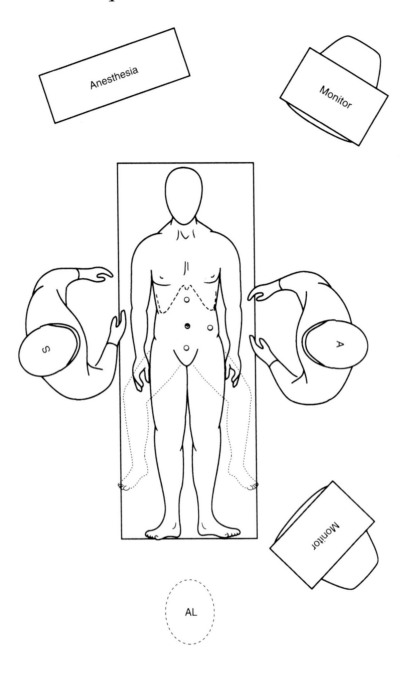

A   Operating room setup for laparoscopic left hemicolectomy. *S*, surgeon; *A*, assistant; *AL*, alternative location for assistant. Note suggested trocar placement.

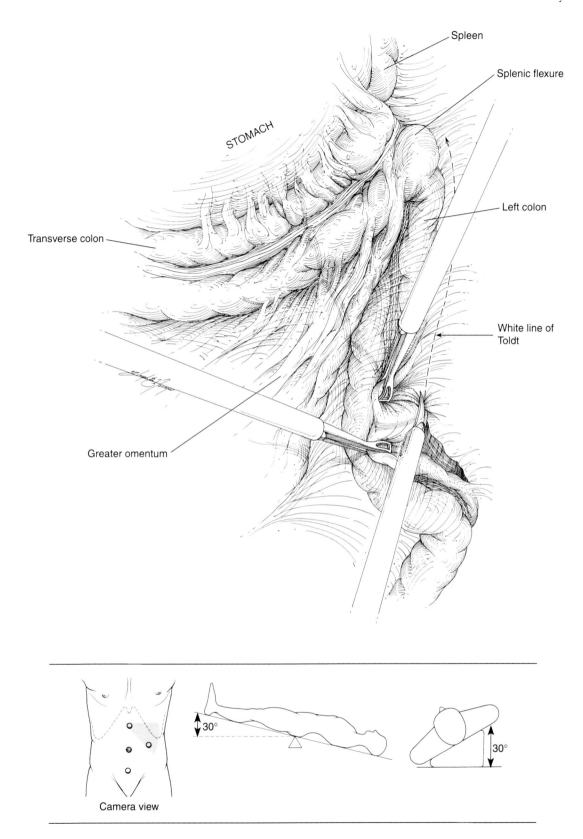

B The peritoneal attachments to the descending colon are sharply incised with cautery scissors from the proximal sigmoid colon to the splenic flexure.

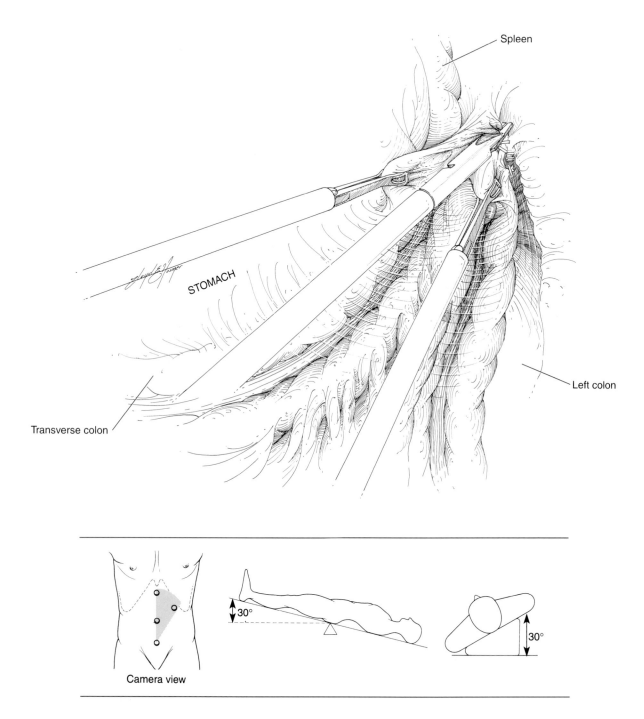

Spleen

STOMACH

Transverse colon

Left colon

Camera view

30°

30°

C When mobilization of the splenic flexure is complete, *there is a shift in the setup:* the patient is placed in reverse Trendelenburg position with a left lateral oblique rotation. A 30-degree laparoscope is placed through the suprapubic trocar. Babcock clamps are used to apply medial and inferior traction to the distal transverse colon and splenic flexure while the splenic flexure is transected between clips.

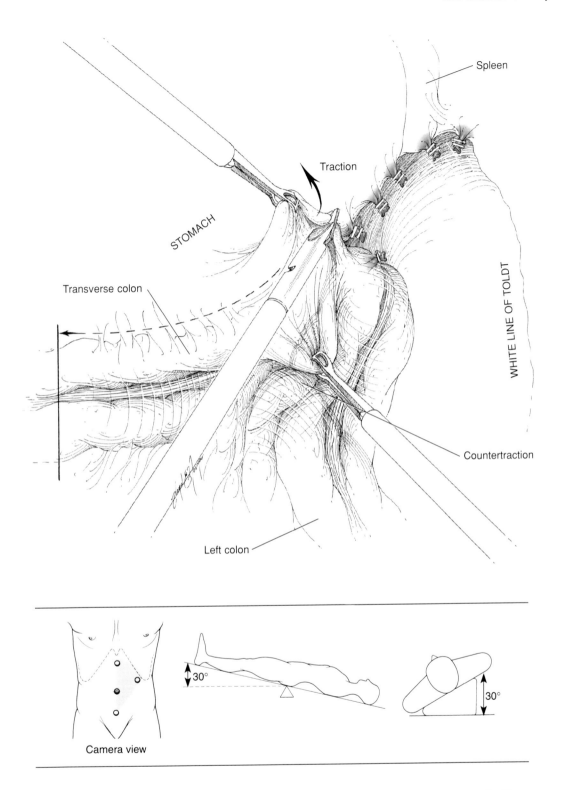

Spleen

Traction

STOMACH

WHITE LINE OF TOLDT

Transverse colon

Countertraction

Left colon

30°

30°

Camera view

D The gastrocolic ligament is transected using cautery scissors and clips. Traction is applied to the superior edge of the gastrocolic ligament while countertraction is directed inferiorly. This continues to the level of the midtransverse colon.

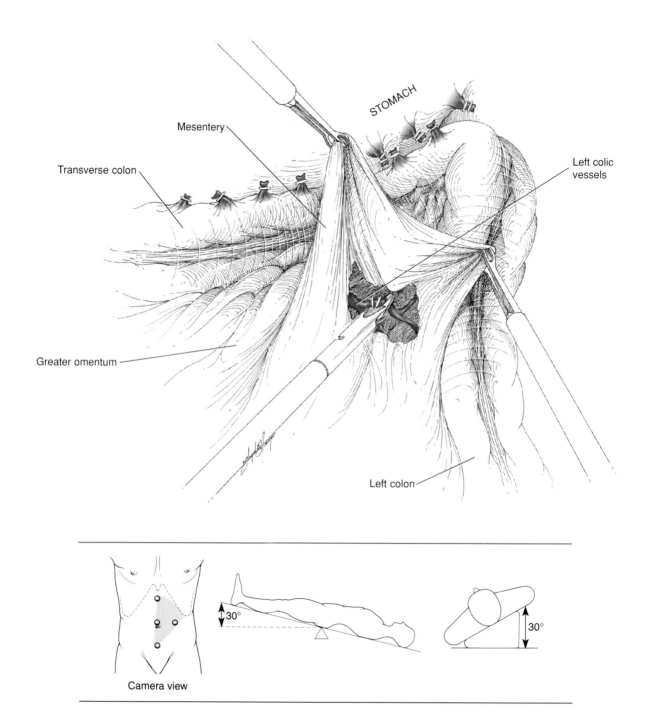

Camera view

E Intracorporeal devascularization. Traction and countertraction are applied to the mesentery after the colon is returned to the normal position. The peritoneal lining over the inferior mesenteric artery (IMA) is incised and the left colic vessels are clipped and transected. After vessel ligation, a mesenteric window is created.

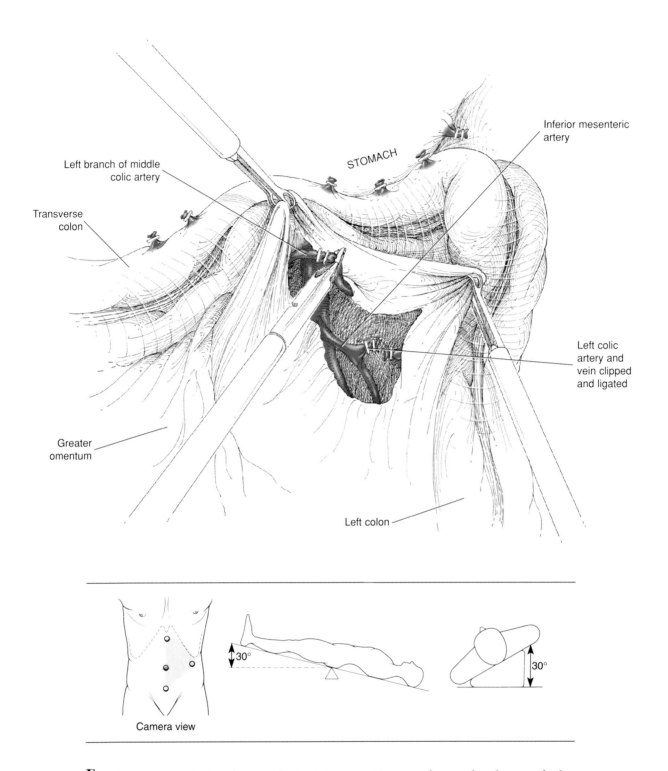

F The mesenteric devascularization continues along the base of the mesentery to the level of the MCA. The left branch of the MCA is carefully identified, clipped, and transected.

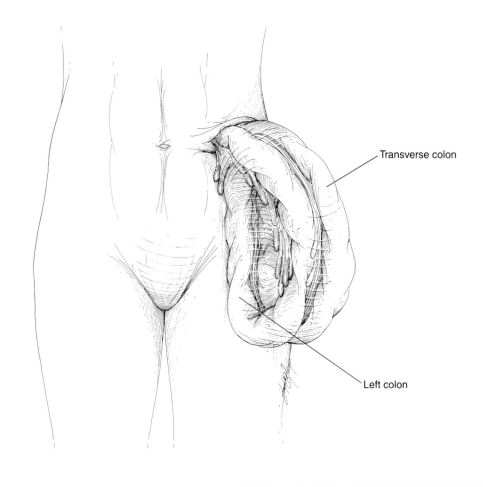

Transverse colon

Left colon

G   After mobilization and devascularization, the left colon is evaluated to determine whether it can reach the anterior abdominal wall without tension. A 4 to 5 mm muscle-splitting incision is made and the specimen is exteriorized.

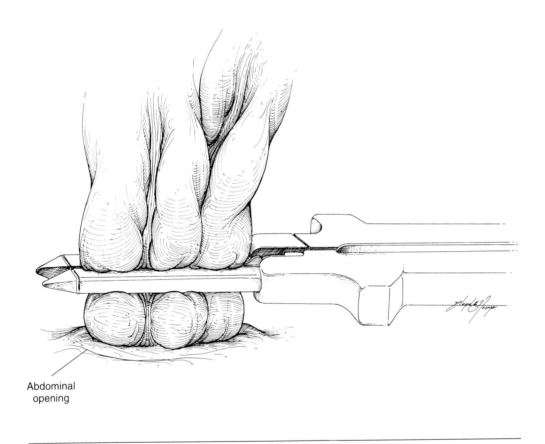

Abdominal
opening

H   The bowel and mesentery are transected with a stapling device, and
the specimen is removed from the field.

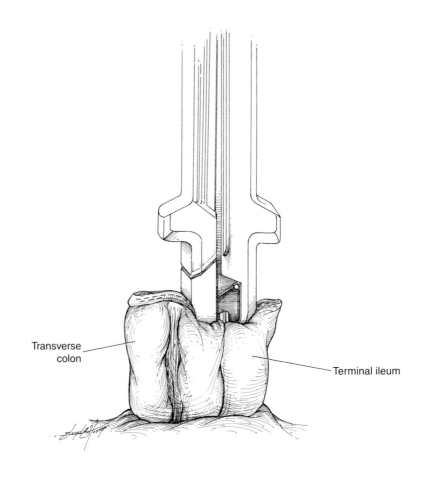

Transverse colon

Terminal ileum

I Side-to-side and functional end-to-end anastomosis created with the stapling device.

8

Sigmoid and Low Anterior Resection

Gustavo Plasencia · Moises Jacobs · Philip F. Caushaj

■

General Considerations

Preoperative Setup and Trocar Placement

Mobilization and Devascularization

Resection and Anastomosis

Intracorporeal Anastomosis

Clinical Caveats

General Considerations

Sigmoid resection and low anterior resection are considered together because, except for the retrorectal and pelvic dissection for the low anterior resection, they are basically performed in a similar manner with similar indications. The most common indications for these procedures are cancer, diverticulitis, and repair of rectal procidentia. Although many advocate that learning laparoscopic techniques occur initially in patients with benign disease, it is important to stress that the pathophysiology of diverticular disease is such that the thickened and foreshortened mesentery may be technically challenging for the novice.

Preoperative Setup and Trocar Placement

The preoperative setup of the operating room and the trocar placement for either laparoscopic sigmoid resection or low anterior resection is the same (Fig. *A*). Two television monitors are positioned at either side of the patient's feet. The surgeon stands to the right of the patient while the camera operator/assistant is to the left of the patient. The patient is placed in a modified lithotomy position. The first trocar is inserted through the umbilicus. The video camera (we prefer a 30-degree angled laparoscope) is initially placed through this umbilical trocar. A diagnostic laparoscopy is performed before the secondary trocars are placed. The second trocar is inserted in the left midclavicular line, approximately two fingerbreadths below the left costal margin. The video camera is subsequently reinserted into this trocar before additional trocars are placed. The third trocar is placed laterally in the anterior axillary line (left flank) at the level of the umbilicus. The fourth trocar is inserted into the suprapubic area.

Mobilization and Devascularization

The surgeon introduces a Babcock clamp through the umbilical trocar to retract the sigmoid colon medially while using cautery scissors through the suprapubic trocar to incise the peritoneal reflection on the left. The assistant directs the video camera through the left upper quadrant trocar and provides additional medial retraction to the sigmoid with a Babcock clamp placed through the left flank trocar. The peritoneal attachments of the sigmoid colon are sharply incised and the sigmoid is reflected superiorly and medially. The pulsation of the iliac artery is visualized and serves as an anatomic landmark for identifying the ureter. Blunt and sharp dissection is performed with a spatula or right-angle clamp inserted through the suprapubic trocar to identify the ureter throughout its course.

Next the mesentery of the sigmoid colon is dissected to expose the underlying blood supply. Superior and lateral traction is applied through the umbilical and flank ports with Babcock clamps placed directly on the mesentery. The inferior mesenteric artery and vein are identified and can be identified anteriorly when appropriate traction is placed on the mesentery (Fig. 8-1). The proper traction bows the mesentery and vessels like violin strings. The surgeon then scores the peritoneum at the root of the mesentery with cautery scissors inserted through the suprapubic port. The small bowel should be retracted from the operative field either with a Babcock clamp directed by the assistant through the flank port or by changing the patient's position. Rarely, a fifth trocar in the mid–right upper quadrant may be necessary and a second assistant, positioned to the right of the surgeon, is needed to retract the small intestine from the pelvis with a fan-type retractor.

Without reflecting the sigmoid colon medially, the surgeon develops the avascular plane proximal to the inferior mesenteric artery (IMA). In-

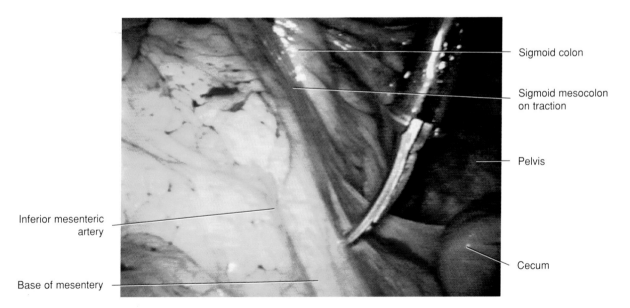

Sigmoid colon

Sigmoid mesocolon on traction

Pelvis

Inferior mesenteric artery

Cecum

Base of mesentery

Fig. 8-1. The mesentery is placed on traction, allowing major vessels to stand out. The peritoneum is scored at the base of the mesentery.

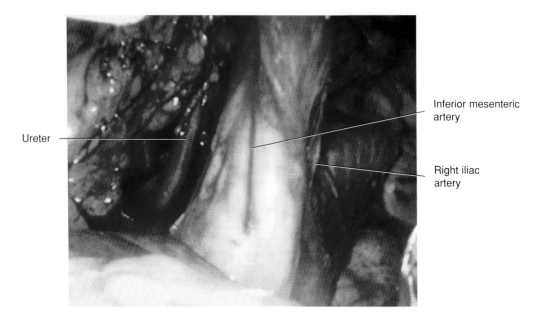

Ureter

Inferior mesenteric
artery

Right iliac
artery

Fig. 8-2. View of ureter through the mesenteric window before division of the inferior mesenteric artery.

spection through this window (Fig. 8-2) allows visualization of the ureter to minimize potential iatrogenic injury to the ureter before IMA ligation. Using careful dissection with right-angled clamps inserted through the suprapubic trocar, the surgeon dissects the IMA free from the inferior mesenteric vein. These vessels are most commonly divided between clips applied through the suprapubic port. If the IMA is considered too large for single clip application, a vascular stapling device or pass-point ligature with a needleless Endo Knot secured extracorporeally may be used to secure the vessel. After the vessels have been ligated, the ureter and iliac artery are once again identified through the window that was created at the base of the mesentery. It is important not to mistake the ureter for a vessel; if there is any doubt before vascular ligation or the ureter is not clearly identified through this mesenteric window, the sigmoid colon should be reflected medially to ensure visualization of the ureter. Blunt dissection continues to the retrorectal space.

Resection and Anastomosis

While the surgeon and assistant continue to apply superior and lateral traction on the mesentery through the umbilical and flank trocars, the distal margin of resection is determined. For a sigmoid colectomy, the distal margin of resection is at the level of the rectosigmoid junction; for a low anterior resection, the distal margin will be at the appropriate level determined by the anatomic location of the lesion. The peritoneal surface of the mesentery is scored with cautery scissors applied through the suprapubic trocar. The devascularization of the mesentery is completed so that the bowel is cleared of mesentery at the distal point of resection. This devascularization is accomplished by electrocautery, clips, or a vascular endolinear stapling device inserted through the suprapubic trocar. This suprapubic trocar is now moved to a 33 mm port.

The endolinear stapling device is applied to the bowel at the distal resection margin and the bowel is transected (Fig. 8-3). By definition, a Hartmann's pouch has been created. The sigmoid colon is delivered through a protective sleeve via the 33 mm trocar site. This incision may occasionally require manual dilation or extension to allow delivery of the bulky colon. The proximal limit of resection is identified and cleared of fat and mesentery. A purse-string suture is applied to the proximal resection line with a mechanical device. The bowel is transected distal to the purse-string (Fig. 8-4). The proximal colon is then sized and, after selecting the appropriate circular stapler size, the surgeon places the anvil and head of the circular stapler in a standard manner. Once the purse-string has been secured, the bowel is returned to the abdominal cavity. The incision is closed and a pneumoperitoneum is reestablished. The intracorporeal anastomosis is then created.

When a low anterior resection is performed, the retrorectal space is entered using blunt and sharp dissection with a spatula, cautery scissors, or a right-angle clamp placed through the suprapubic trocar. This dissection proceeds caudally to Waldeyer's fascia. To complete the retrorectal dissection and expose the levator ani, Waldeyer's fascia must be completely incised.

The anterior rectovesicular peritoneal investiture is now incised with cautery scissors placed through the suprapubic trocar while superior traction of the peritoneum is accomplished by a Babcock clamp placed in the left flank trocar. The surgeon maintains cranioinferior traction to the rectum by a Babcock clamp inserted through the umbilical trocar. After the anterior rectovesicular peritoneal investiture has been fully incised, blunt dissection is used to develop the plane between the anterior surface of the rectum and the prostate (or vagina). This dissection should be continued to the level of the levator ani anteriorly.

The uterus may occasionally obscure the view of the lower pelvis; consequently, uterine manipulations may be necessary to provide anterior retraction of the uterus. However, the Babcock clamp retracting the peritoneal lining of the rectovesicular investiture will also lift the uterus from

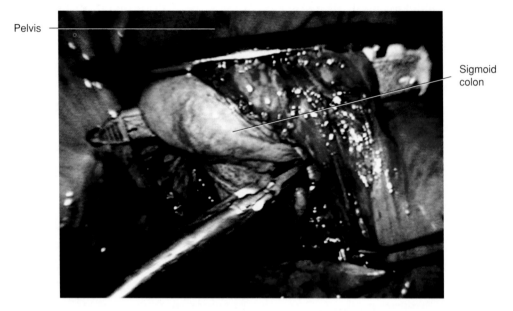

Pelvis

Sigmoid colon

Fig. 8-3. Transection of the sigmoid colon with an endostapler.

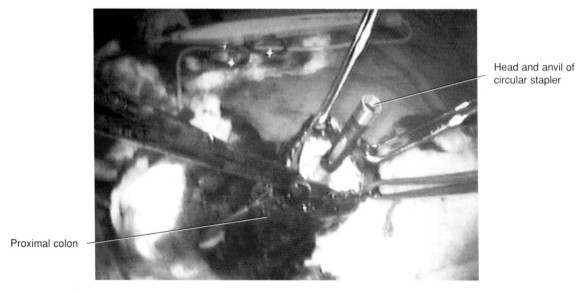

Head and anvil of circular stapler

Proximal colon

Fig. 8-4. Placement of the head and anvil of the circular stapler in the proximal colon.

the operative field. The lateral stalks are then easily identified and developed and divided between clips applied through the suprapubic trocar. The specimen side of the lateral stalks is cauterized to establish hemostasis.

Clips should not be placed on the specimen side of the rectum to prevent malfunction of the endolinear stapling device. The surgeon must take care to not "cone down" on the rectum during mobilization; this could have disastrous consequences in operations performed for malignancy, as it does in standard open surgery of the rectum. We are careful to resect the entire mesorectum in continuity before bowel transection. The 10/12 mm suprapubic trocar is then replaced with a 33 mm trocar so that the stapling device can be inserted.

Once the rectum is fully mobilized, the anatomic location of the lesion is verified endoscopically and the distal resection margin is determined. The stapling device is positioned at the distal point of resection. After the stapler has been properly positioned, it is important to ensure that the ureter has not been trapped within the jaws of the stapling device. The stapler is then fired. A Hartmann's pouch has now been created.

An incision is then made incorporating the previously made trocar site for the 33 mm suprapubic trocar, and the proximal bowel is delivered through this incision. We routinely use a plastic sleeve to protect the incision from potential contamination. The proximal margin of resection is selected and cleared of fat and mesentery. A mechanical purse-string suture is applied to the proximal margin of resection. The bowel is then resected extracorporeally. The proximal colon is then sized. After selecting the appropriate circular stapler size, the surgeon places the anvil and head of the circular stapler in the proximal colon and the purse-string is securely tied. The proximal bowel is returned to the abdominal cavity. The incision is sealed around the 33 mm trocar with towel clips and a pneumoperitoneum is reestablished.

Intracorporeal Anastomosis

The shaft of the circular stapling device is passed transanally and the spearhead is extruded through the Hartmann's staple line (Fig. 8-6). This process is aided by applying countertraction, with a Babcock clamp placed through the suprapubic trocar, along the staple line of the rectum. The surgeon and assistant orient the head and anvil with the shaft; this is easily accomplished by placing proximal traction on the colon by grasping the colon proximal to the stapler head with a Babcock clamp through the umbilical trocar and then grasping the exposed center rod of the anvil with either a Babcock clamp or any instrument devised to facilitate this placed through the suprapubic trocar. When union between the anvil and shaft has been accomplished, the circular stapler is closed (Fig. 8-5).

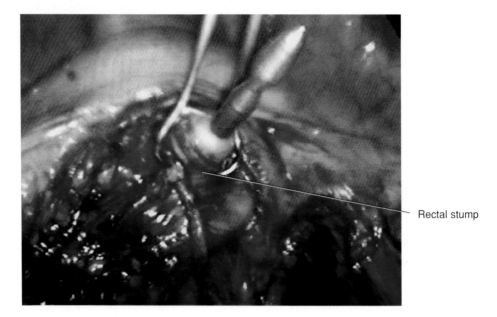

Rectal stump

Fig. 8-5. Passage of the spear of the circular stapler through the distal staple line.

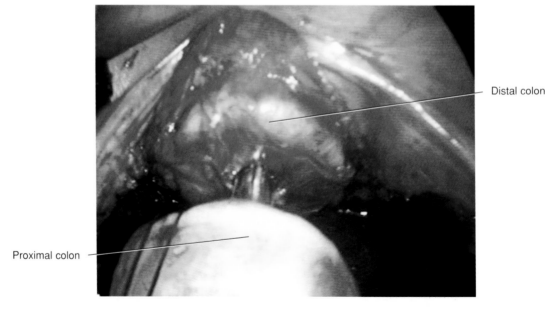

Distal colon

Proximal colon

Fig. 8-6. Closing of both ends of the circular stapler.

If excess tension is evident before the anastomosis is created, additional mobilization of the peritoneal attachments of the descending colon may be necessary, including takedown of the splenic flexure.

If the splenic flexure must be taken down, one of the television monitors must be moved to the head of the patient on the left. The assistant subsequently moves between the patient's legs. The video camera is switched to the suprapubic trocar, and mobilization of the splenic flexure proceeds as described in Chapter 7.

After a tension-free anastomosis is ensured, the stapling device is fired and an intracorporeal double-stapled end-to-end anastomosis is created. If there is a question regarding tissue approximation, the camera should be switched to a suprapubic trocar to change the field of view before the stapling device is fired. The firing of the stapler automatically cuts the purse-string suture.

The "doughnuts" are visually inspected and the integrity of the anastomosis is tested by insufflating air through a sigmoidoscope passed transanally while the anastomosis is submerged in saline. The proximal bowel should be occluded to facilitate this maneuver. In the case of a low anterior resection, a drain is placed via the left lateral trocar site into the pelvis. The left lower quadrant and trocar incisions are then closed.

If an anastomotic leak is demonstrated by the technique just described, the surgeon has several options: direct intracorporeal suture repair of a small anterior defect; extending the suprapubic incision in a transverse fashion for a directed open repair; transanal repair if the anastomosis is low and near the anal canal; proximal diverting ostomy; and conversion to an open procedure. The experience and intraoperative judgment of the surgeon will dictate the correct option.

Clinical Caveats

- During the mobilization and devascularization phase of laparoscopic sigmoid resection and low anterior resection, the pulsation of the iliac artery serves as an anatomic landmark for the identification of the ureter.

- An avascular plane developed proximally to the inferior mesenteric artery allows visualization of the ureter before vascular ligation. This serves as an important safeguard to minimize iatrogenic injury to the ureter.

- During a low anterior resection, the retrorectal space is preferably entered with cautery dissection. Excellent hemostasis should be the hallmark of the pelvic dissection.

- When performing low anterior resection laparoscopically, the surgeon should avoid "coning down" of the rectal mesentery. This could minimize the potential for inadequate cancer surgery.

Surgical Technique

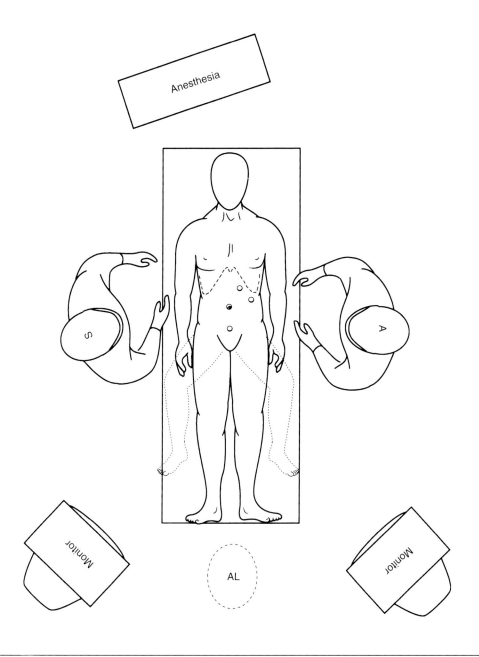

A   Operating room setup for sigmoid and low anterior resection. *S*, surgeon; *A*, assistant, *AL*, alternative location for assistant. Note suggested trocar placement.

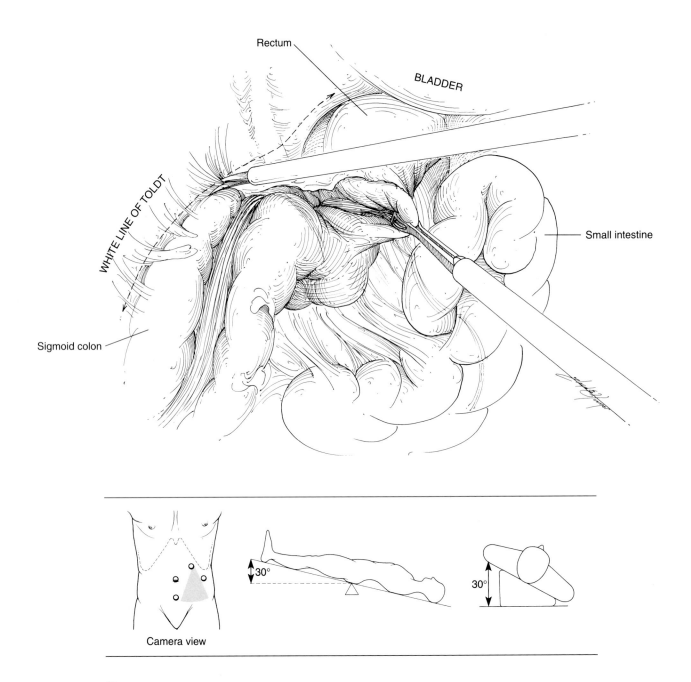

B   The surgeon places traction on the sigmoid colon medially with a Babcock clamp through the umbilical trocar while incising the peritoneal attachments with cautery scissors through the suprapubic trocar.

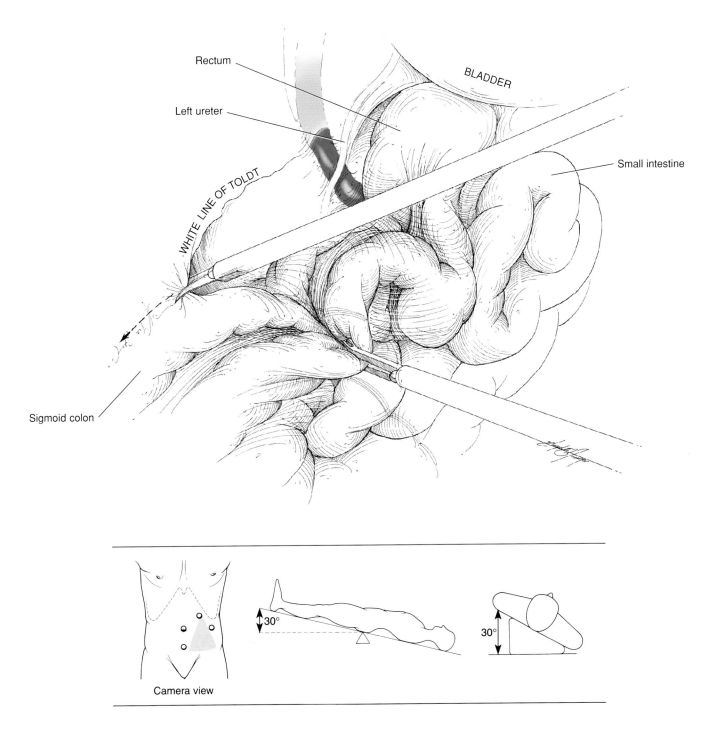

C   The ureter must be identified before vascular ligation is performed.

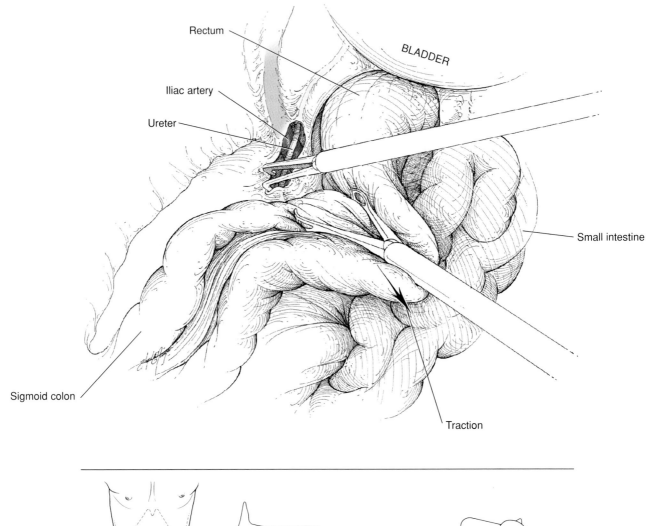

Rectum

Iliac artery

Ureter

BLADDER

Small intestine

Sigmoid colon

Traction

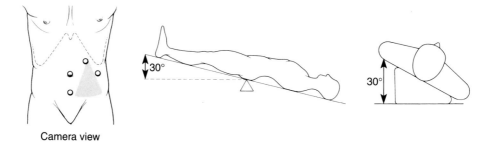

Camera view

30°

30°

D Visualization of the pulsation of the artery serves as an anatomic landmark in identifying the ureter. Dissection is performed with a right-angle clamp through the suprapubic trocar to identify the ureter throughout its course.

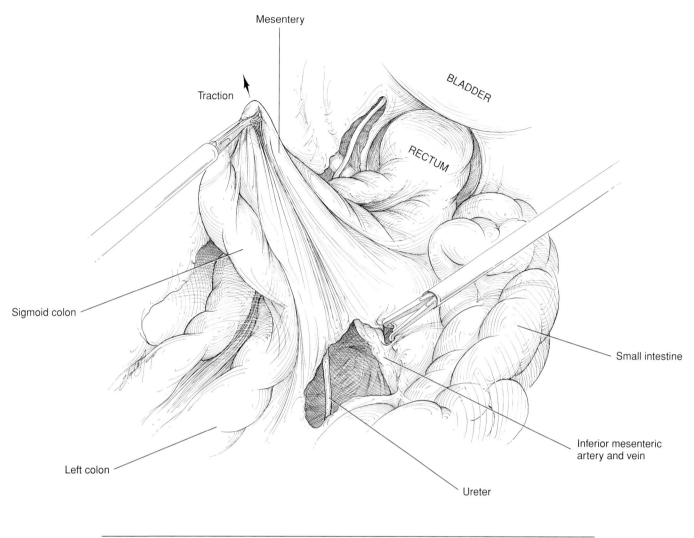

Mesentery

Traction

BLADDER

RECTUM

Sigmoid colon

Small intestine

Inferior mesenteric
artery and vein

Left colon

Ureter

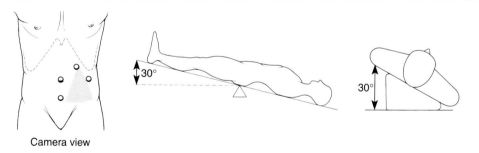

Camera view

30°

30°

E   A Babcock clamp inserted through the umbilical trocar is used to apply superior traction to the mesentery. The peritoneum at the base of
the vessels is incised and the inferior mesenteric vessels are separated.

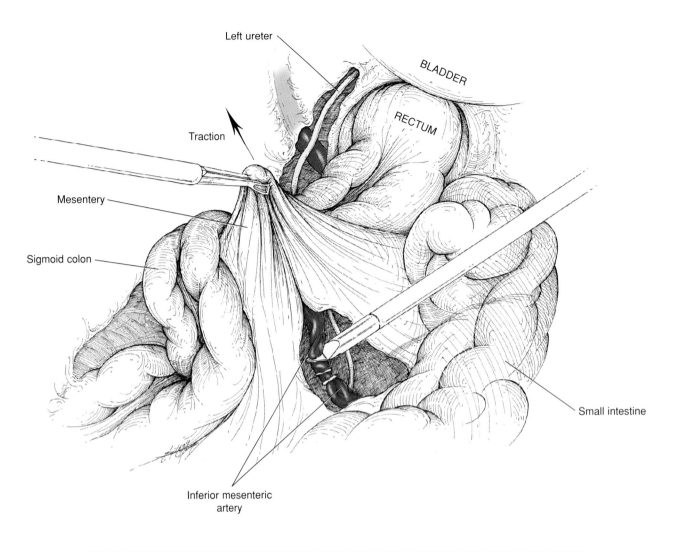

Left ureter

BLADDER

RECTUM

Traction

Mesentery

Sigmoid colon

Small intestine

Inferior mesenteric
artery

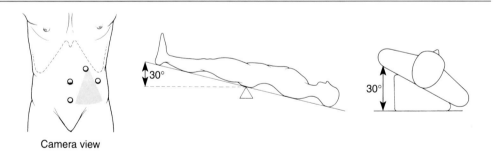

Camera view

30°

30°

F   The mesenteric vessels are individually ligated with a clip applier inserted through the suprapubic trocar.

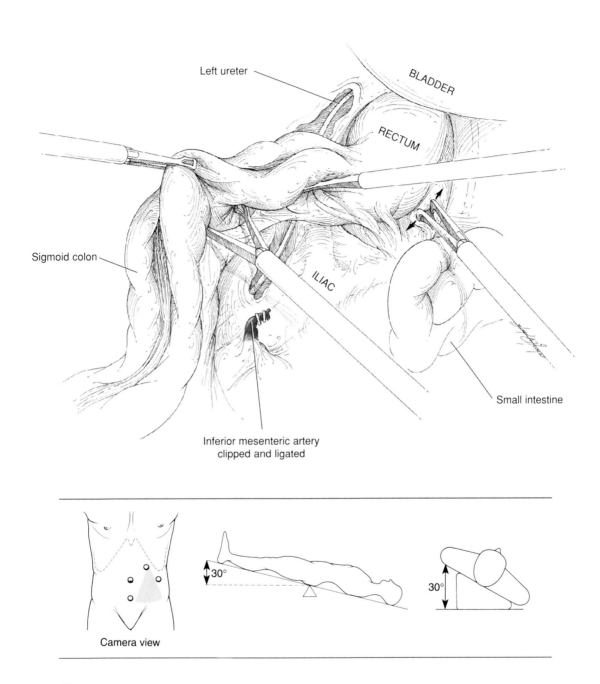

G   The entire course of the left ureter is exposed.

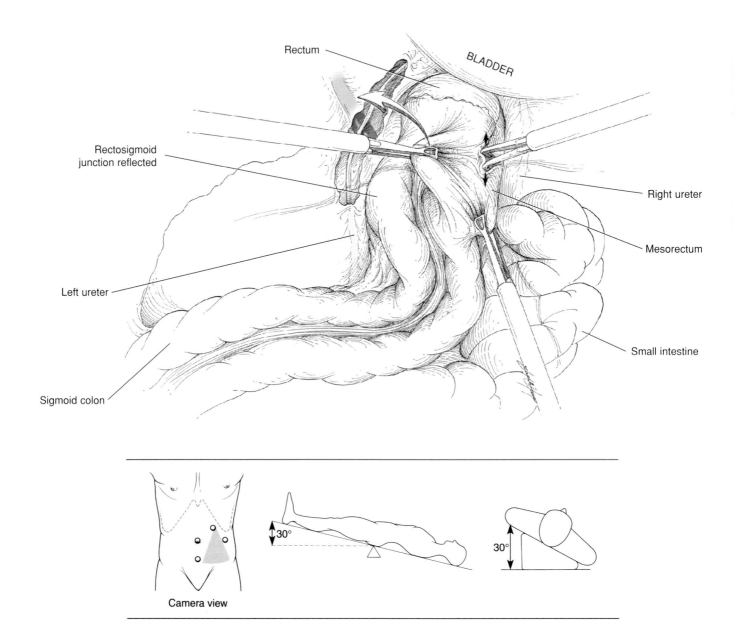

Rectum

BLADDER

Rectosigmoid
junction reflected

Right ureter

Mesorectum

Left ureter

Small intestine

Sigmoid colon

Camera view

30°

30°

H The lateral stalks are easily identified and developed by the surgeon
with a right-angle clamp inserted through the suprapubic trocar. The
assistant applies traction to the rectum superiorly and laterally and
countertraction is directed medially via the umbilical trocar.

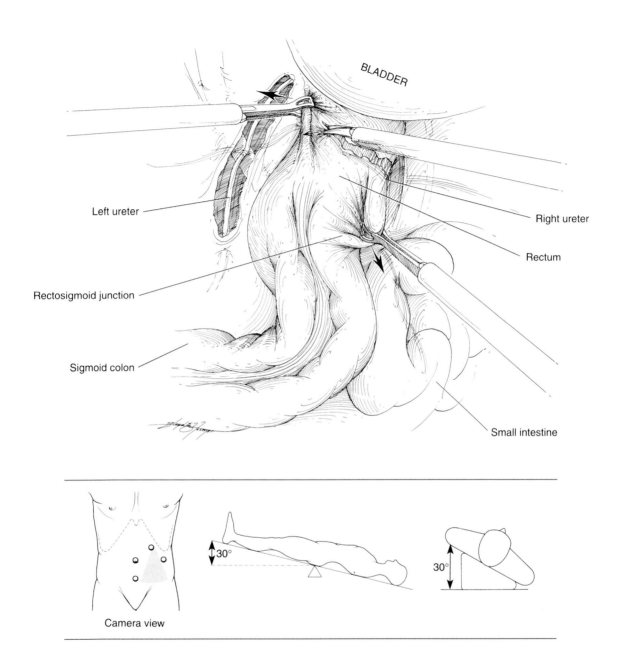

BLADDER

Left ureter

Right ureter

Rectosigmoid junction

Rectum

Sigmoid colon

Small intestine

Camera view

30°

30°

I   The anterior rectovesicular peritoneal investiture is sharply incised with cautery scissors through the suprapubic trocar.

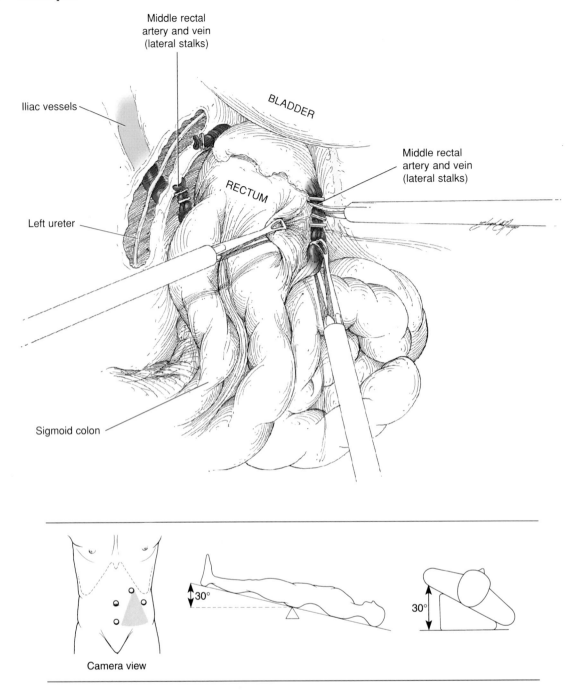

Middle rectal
artery and vein
(lateral stalks)

Iliac vessels

BLADDER

Middle rectal
artery and vein
(lateral stalks)

Left ureter

RECTUM

Sigmoid colon

Camera view

30°

30°

J   Lateral stalks are clipped and transected. Clips and cautery scissors are
applied through the suprapubic trocar.

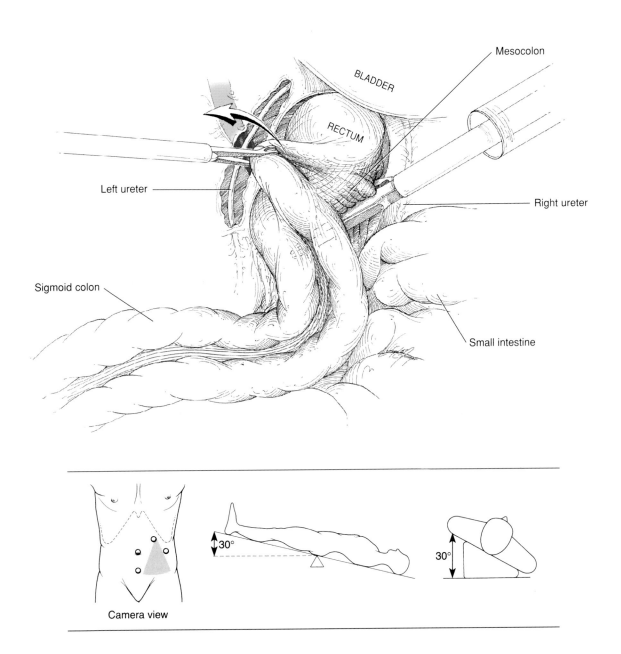

K The rectum is retracted superiorly by an endolinear stapler inserted through the suprapubic trocar.

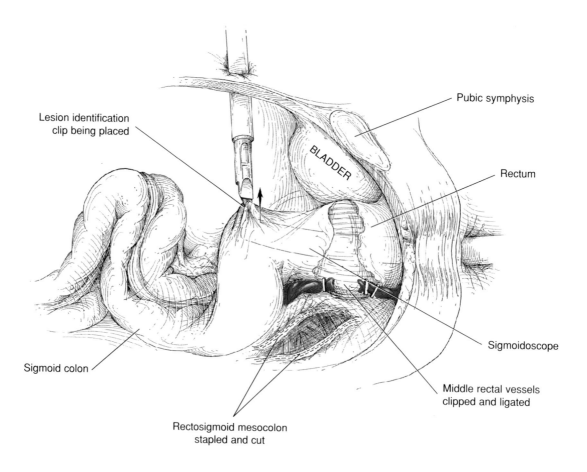

Lesion identification
clip being placed

Pubic symphysis

BLADDER

Rectum

Sigmoid colon

Sigmoidoscope

Middle rectal vessels
clipped and ligated

Rectosigmoid mesocolon
stapled and cut

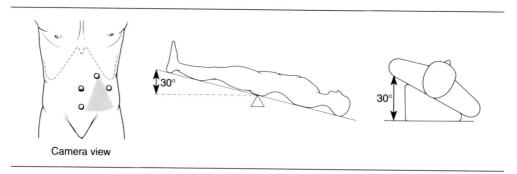

30°

30°

Camera view

L   The lesion is located by sigmoidoscopy and marked with a clip to ensure proper margins.

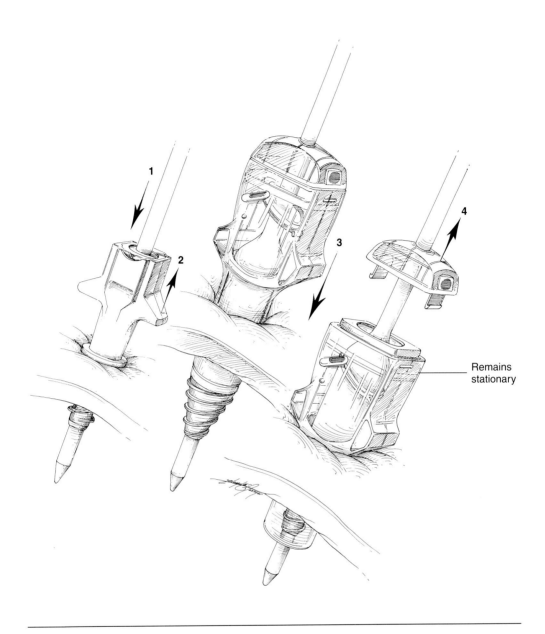

Remains
stationary

M Conversion of the suprapubic trocar to a 33 mm trocar. Step 1, an exchange rod is inserted into the existing trocar. Step 2, the 12 mm trocar is removed, leaving the exchange rod. Step 3, after extending the skin incision, the 33 mm trocar is inserted over the exchange rod. Step 4, the exchange rod and insert are removed, leaving the 33 mm trocar.

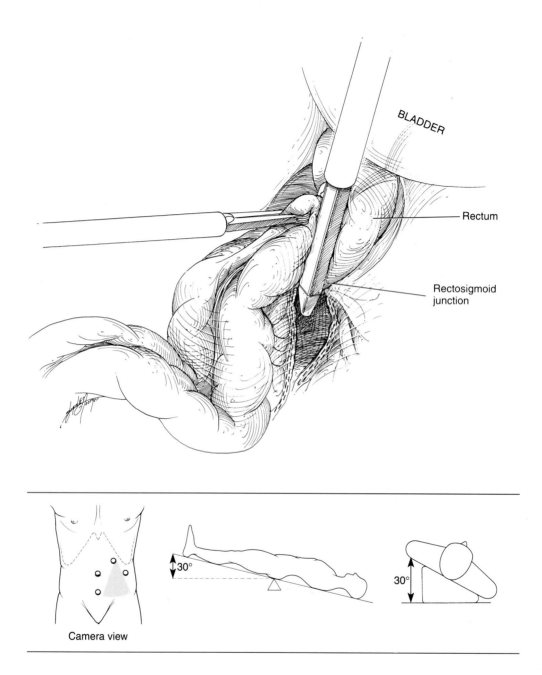

N   The endolinear stapler is positioned at the distal margin of the mobilized rectum. This stapler is inserted through the suprapubic 33 mm trocar.

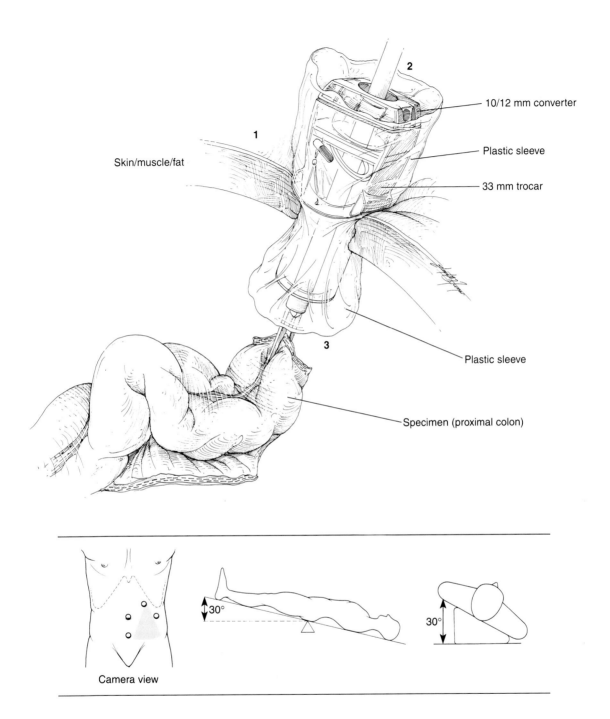

10/12 mm converter

Plastic sleeve

33 mm trocar

Skin/muscle/fat

Plastic sleeve

Specimen (proximal colon)

Camera view

30°

30°

O   A protective wound barrier is positioned and the specimen is grasped by a Babcock clamp before delivery of the specimen through the 33 mm trocar.

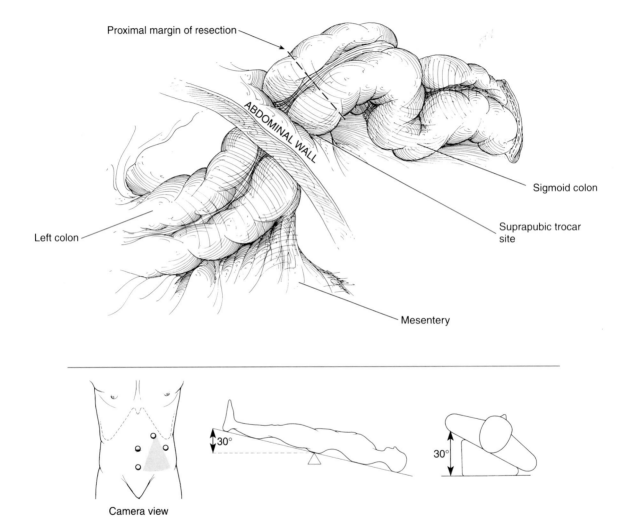

Proximal margin of resection

ABDOMINAL WALL

Sigmoid colon

Left colon

Suprapubic trocar site

Mesentery

Camera view

30°

30°

P   The specimen is delivered intracorporeally and the proximal margin is identified.

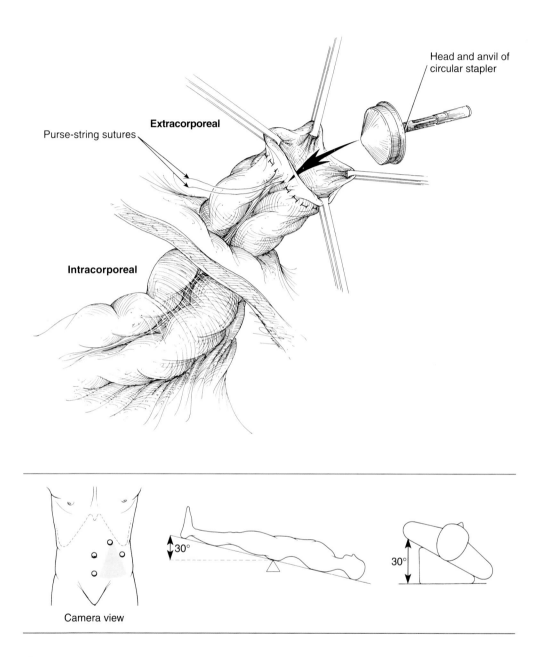

Head and anvil of circular stapler

Extracorporeal

Purse-string sutures

Intracorporeal

Camera view

30°

30°

Q   The bowel is resected and purse-string sutures are applied in preparation for the head and anvil of the circular stapler.

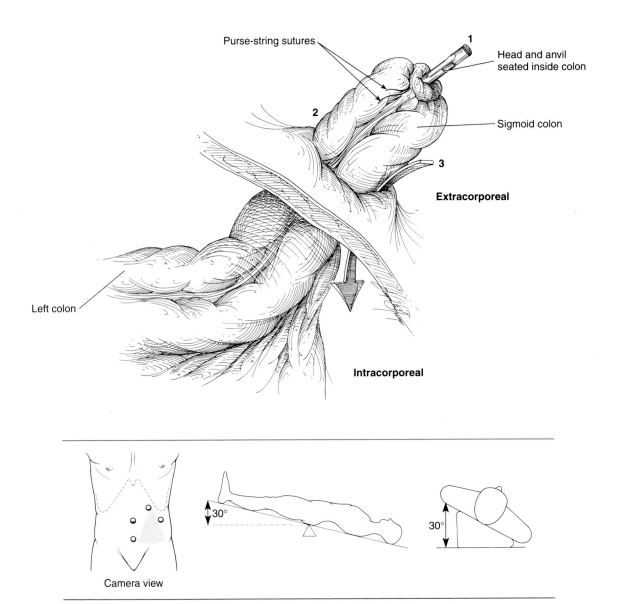

R   Purse-string sutures are secured around the head and anvil of the circular stapler. Step 1, seat the trocar in the colon; step 2, tie purse-string sutures; step 3, push the colon back into the abdomen.

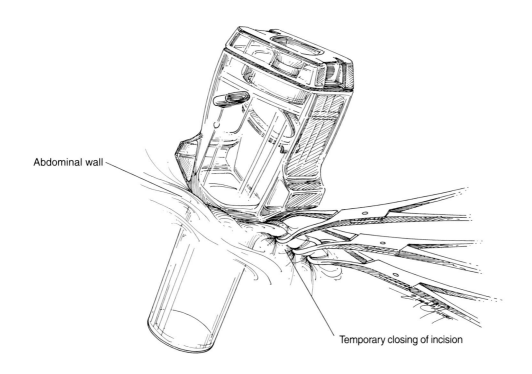

Abdominal wall

Temporary closing of incision

S   The proximal colon is returned to the abdominal cavity with the head and anvil inserted. The 33 mm trocar is reinserted into the previous trocar site. The remaining excess incision length is approximated with towel clips to ensure adequate seal for reinduction of the pneumoperitoneum.

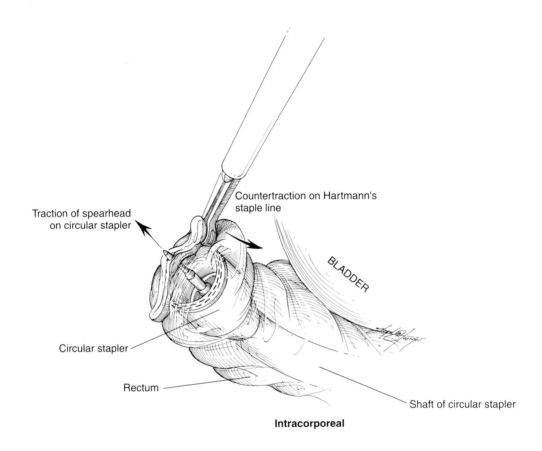

Intracorporeal

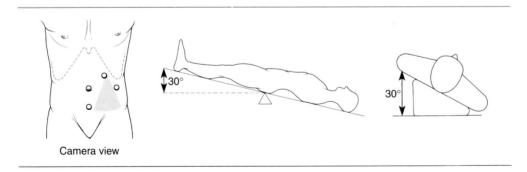

Camera view

30°

30°

T   The shaft of the circular stapler is passed transanally and the spearhead is extruded through the Hartmann's pouch. This process is facilitated by applying countertraction through a Babcock clamp placed through the suprapubic trocar along the staple line and rectum.

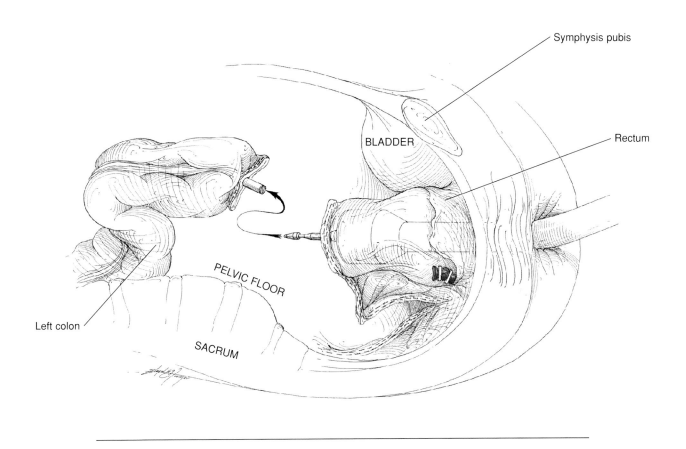

U   Cross-sectional view demonstrating insertion of the stapling device.

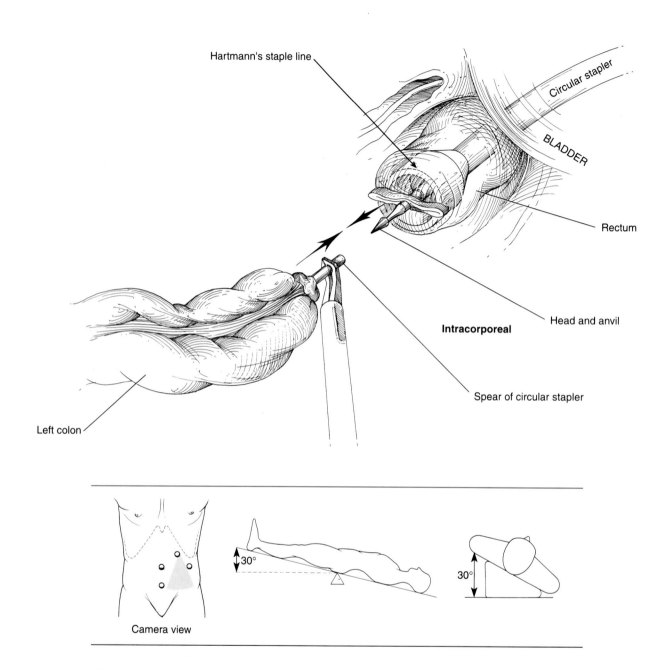

Hartmann's staple line

Circular stapler

BLADDER

Rectum

Head and anvil

Intracorporeal

Spear of circular stapler

Left colon

30°

30°

Camera view

V The surgeon orients the head and anvil with an instrument specifical-
ly devised for this purpose. An assistant stabilizes the shaft of the stapler to facilitate union.

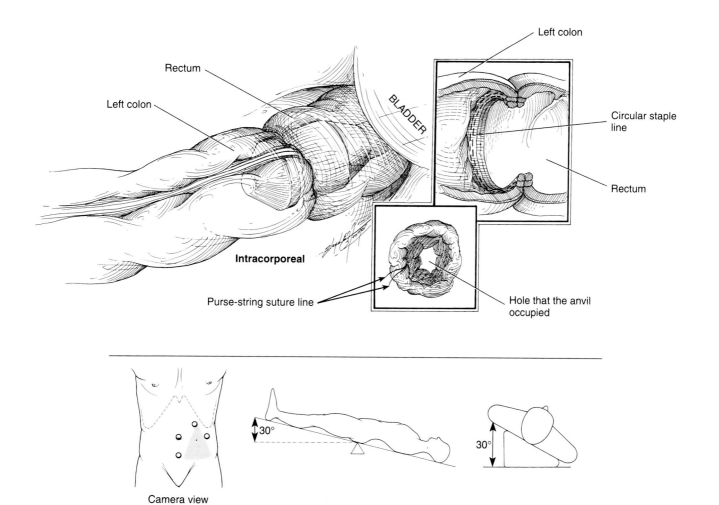

Rectum

Left colon

BLADDER

Intracorporeal

Purse-string suture line

Left colon

Circular staple line

Rectum

Hole that the anvil occupied

Camera view

30°

30°

W The stapler is closed and fired. The "doughnuts" are examined for integrity of the anastomosis. *Upper inset:* Sagittal view of the completed anastomosis. *Lower inset:* Specimen made from circular cutter.

9

Abdominoperineal Resection

Morris Franklin ▪ Moises Jacobs ▪ Gustavo Plasencia ▪
Philip F. Caushaj

General Considerations

Preoperative Setup and Trocar Placement

Mobilization and Devascularization

Resection and Colostomy Formation

Clinical Caveats

General Considerations

Abdominoperineal resection (APR) is often performed for distal rectal cancer. It is also indicated for proctectomy for severe irritable bowel disease. The prevalence of sphincter-preserving options has relegated the role of abdominoperineal resection to a procedure of last choice. The most important consideration for APR for malignancy is to obtain appropriate lateral margins and to completely resect the mesorectum. Interestingly, laparoscopic technique offers an exceptional view of the pelvis to the levators. This laparoscopic approach may be superior to conventional APR; however, further experience with the approach will be necessary to determine whether this is true.

Preoperative Setup and Trocar Placement

The operating room setup and trocar placement are the same for APR as for laparoscopic sigmoid resection or low anterior resection (see Chapter 8). The colostomy site is premarked in the left lower quadrant of the abdomen by the enterostomal therapist. Early in our experience, we inserted the left lateral trocar through the anticipated colostomy site; however, we noted that this trocar placement was too close to the other trocar sites. This close proximity limited the operative field of view and diminished our ability to maneuver and dissect through the other trocars. The patient is always placed in a modified lithotomy position. Rectal irrigations and colonoscopy can be performed at the surgeon's discretion. The surgeon and assistant are positioned as for the sigmoid and low anterior resection.

The surgeon uses the suprapubic and umbilical trocars exclusively during the procedure; the video camera is directed through the left upper quadrant trocar. The assistant retracts the bowel or mesentery through the left flank port. The first trocar is inserted through the umbilicus. The video camera (we prefer a 30-degree angled scope) is initially placed through this umbilical port. A diagnostic laparoscopy is performed before secondary trocars are placed. The second trocar is inserted in the midclavicular line, approximately two fingerbreadths below the left costal margin. The video camera is subsequently reinserted into this trocar before additional trocars are placed. Subsequently the third trocar is placed laterally in the anterior axillary line (left flank) at the level of the umbilicus. The fourth trocar is inserted into the suprapubic area.

Mobilization and Devascularization

The surgeon introduces a Babcock clamp through the umbilical trocar to retract the sigmoid colon medially while using cautery scissors through the suprapubic trocar to incise the peritoneal reflection on the left. The assistant directs the camera through the left upper quadrant trocar and provides additional medial retraction to the sigmoid with a Babcock clamp through the left flank trocar. The peritoneal attachments of the sigmoid colon are sharply incised and the sigmoid colon is reflected medially (Fig. 9-1). The pulsation of the iliac artery is visualized and serves as an anatomic landmark for identification of the ureter. Blunt and sharp dissection with a spatula or a right-angled clamp inserted through the suprapubic trocar is performed to identify the ureter throughout its course.

The mesentery of the sigmoid colon is now dissected to expose the underlying blood supply. Superior and lateral traction is applied through the umbilical and flank ports with Babcock clamps placed directly on the mesentery. The inferior mesenteric artery and vein are identified. The proper traction bows the mesentery and vessels like violin strings. The surgeon then scores the peritoneum at the root of the mesentery with cautery scissors inserted through the suprapubic port. The small bowel should be retracted from the operative field, either by means of a Babcock clamp di-

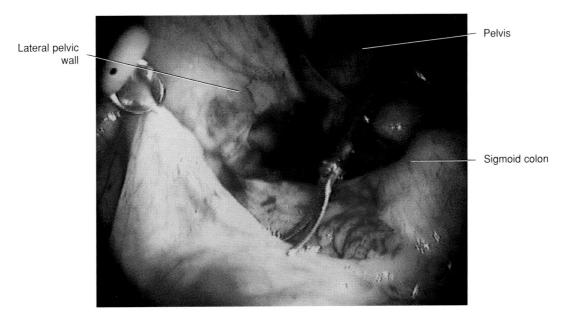

Fig. 9-1. Mobilization of the rectosigmoid junction.

rected by the assistant through the flank trocar or by changing the patient's position. Rarely, a fifth trocar in the mid–right upper quadrant is necessary and a second assistant, positioned to the right of the surgeon, is needed to retract the small intestine from the pelvis with a fan-type retractor.

Without reflecting the sigmoid colon medially, the surgeon develops the avascular plane proximal to the inferior mesenteric artery is developed. Inspection through this window allows visualization of the ureter to minimize the potential for iatrogenic injury to the ureter before ligation of the inferior mesenteric artery. Using careful dissection with right-angled clamps inserted through the suprapubic port, the IMA is dissected free from the inferior mesenteric vein. These vessels are most commonly divided between clips applied through the suprapubic port. If the inferior mesenteric artery is considered too large for single clip application, a vascular stapling device or pass-point ligature with a needleless Endoknot secured extracorporeally should be used to secure the vessel. After the vessels have been ligated, the ureter and iliac artery are once again identified through the window that has been created at the base of the mesentery. It is important not to mistake the ureter for a vessel. If there is any doubt before vascular ligation or the ureter is not clearly seen through this mesenteric window, the sigmoid colon should be reflected medially to ensure visualization of the ureter. Blunt dissection then continues to the retrorectal space.

Resection and Colostomy Formation

While the surgeon and assistant apply superior and lateral traction on the mesentery through the umbilical and flank trocars, the retrorectal space is dissected with spatula, cautery scissors, or right-angled clamp placed through the suprapubic port. This dissection proceeds caudally to Waldeyer's fascia. To complete the retrorectal dissection and expose the levator ani, Waldeyer's fascia must be completely incised.

The anterior rectovesicular peritoneal investiture is now incised with cautery scissors placed through the suprapubic trocar while the peritoneum is retracted superiorly by means of a Babcock clamp placed in a left flank trocar. The surgeon maintains cranioinferior traction on the rectum by a Babcock clamp inserted through the umbilical port. After the anterior rectovesicular peritoneal investiture has been fully incised, blunt dissection is used to develop the plane between the anterior surface of the rectum and the prostate (or vagina). This dissection should be continued to the level of the levator ani anteriorly. The uterus may occasionally obscure the view of the lower pelvis; consequently, uterine manipulations may be necessary to provide anterior retraction of the uterus. However, the Babcock clamp retracting the peritoneal lining of the rectovesicular investiture will also lift the uterus from the operative field.

The lateral stalks are then easily identified and developed and divided between clips applied through the suprapubic trocar. The surgeon must be cautious to not "cone down" on the rectum during the mobilization. This could potentially have disastrous consequences in operations performed for malignancy, as occurs in standard open surgery of the rectum as well.

Once the rectum is fully mobilized, the surgeon turns to the division of the marginal artery and clearance of the mesenteric tissue at the proximal margin of resection of the colon. Through the suprapubic trocar, a 35 or 60 mm stapling device is inserted and positioned at the proximal resection margin after converting to an 18 mm trocar. The stapler is then fired and the bowel transected (Fig. 9-2). The proximal bowel is grasped by a Babcock clamp inserted through the suprapubic port and is presented to the peritoneal side of the previously marked stoma site. At this juncture, the stoma is created externally in the usual manner. After the posterior fascia is opened, the pneumoperitoneum is lost; however, with a Babcock clamp placed externally through the stoma site, the proximal bowel is grasped and delivered extracorporeally. The excess bowel is resected to skin level and the colostomy matured.

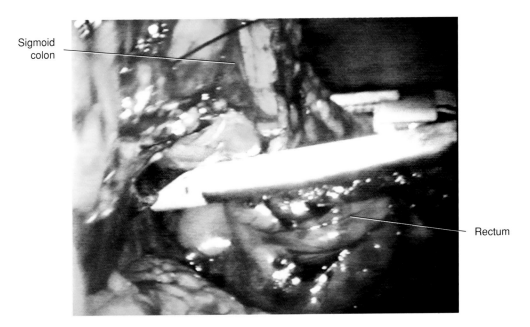

Fig. 9-2. Transecting the sigmoid colon in an abdominoperineal resection using a vascular endostapler.

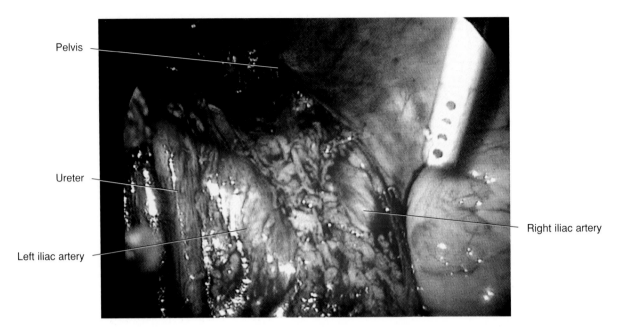

Pelvis

Ureter

Left iliac artery

Right iliac artery

Fig. 9-3. View of the retroperitoneum during abdominoperineal resection.

The perineal resection is performed in the usual fashion. An elliptic incision is made around the anus (see Fig. Q, p. 168). This dissection is carried out proximally until the abdominal and perineal planes are met and the rectum is completely freed from its attachments (Fig. 9-3). The specimen is removed through the perineum. After obtaining adequate hemostasis, the perineal defect and skin are closed. Once the perineum is closed, the abdominal cavity is reinsufflated with CO_2, the pneumoperitoneum is reestablished, and hemostasis is evaluated. If postoperative radiation therapy is being considered, a pelvic sling with Vicryl mesh may be used; otherwise, the peritoneum is not usually reapproximated. A closed suction drain is placed into the pelvis through the left lateral trocar site. All trocar sites are then closed.

Clinical Caveats

- When performing laparoscopic abdominoperineal resection, be careful to obtain appropriate oncologic margins laterally as well as complete mesorectal resections.

- If you are using ureteral stents to facilitate identification of the ureter, be mindful that the ureteral stents may bow the ureters out of their traditional domain and may actually precipitate an injury.

- The perineal surgery is performed in the usual manner. However, the laparoscopic mobilization anteriorly should be completed before the perineal and abdominal surgeons "meet."

- If postoperative radiation is to be performed, then use of an absorbable mesh should be considered.

Surgical Technique

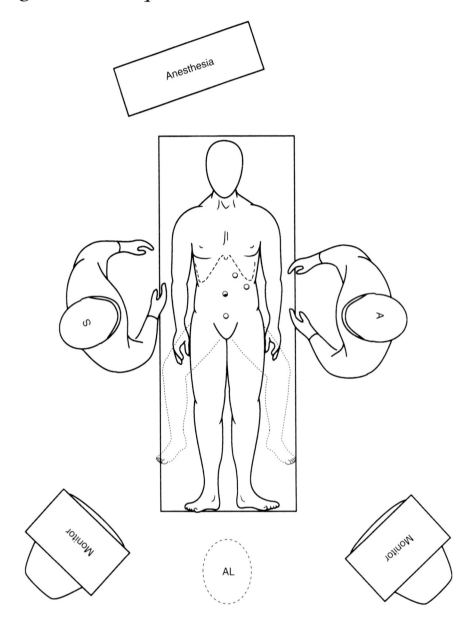

A   Operating room setup for sigmoid and low anterior resection. *S,* surgeon; *A,* assistant, *AL,* alternative location for assistant. Note suggested trocar placement.

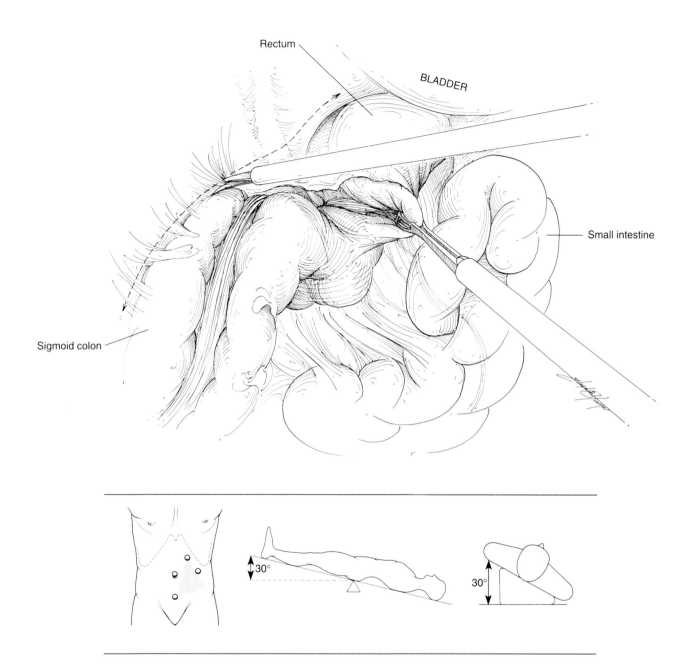

B   The surgeon places traction on the sigmoid colon medially with a Babcock clamp through the umbilical trocar while incising the peritoneal attachments with cautery scissors through the suprapubic trocar.

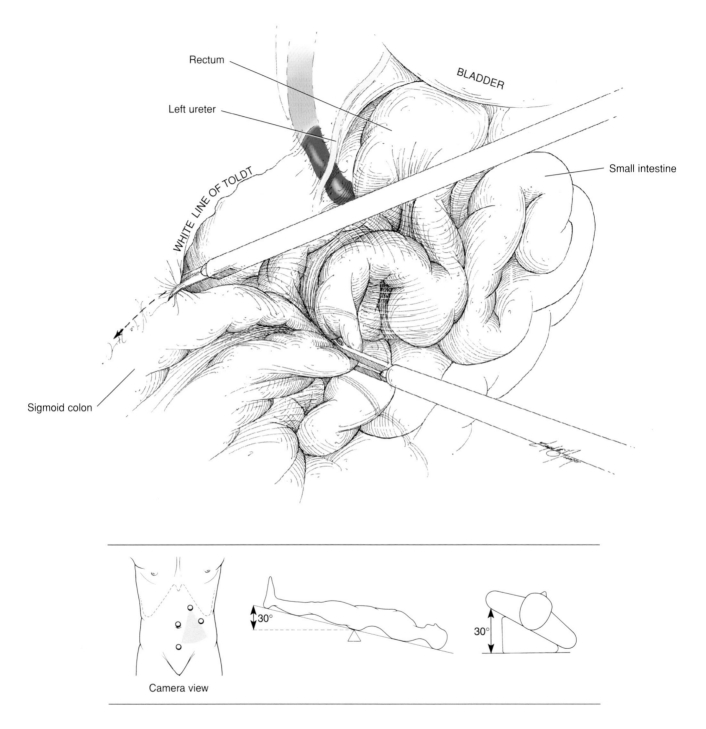

Rectum

Left ureter

BLADDER

WHITE LINE OF TOLDT

Small intestine

Sigmoid colon

Camera view

30°

30°

C The ureter must be identified before vascular ligation is performed.

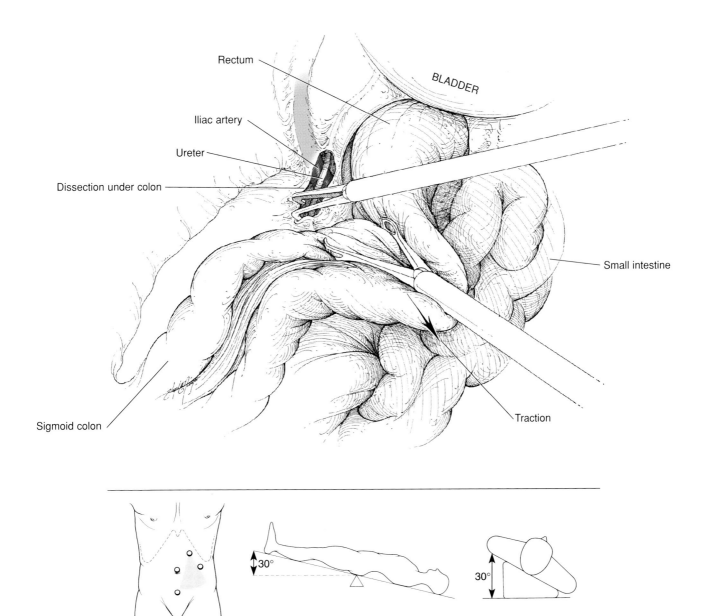

Rectum

BLADDER

Iliac artery

Ureter

Dissection under colon

Small intestine

Sigmoid colon

Traction

Camera view

30°

30°

D   Visualization of the pulsation of the artery serves as an anatomic landmark in identifying the ureter. Dissection is performed with a right-angle clamp through the suprapubic trocar to identify the ureter throughout its course.

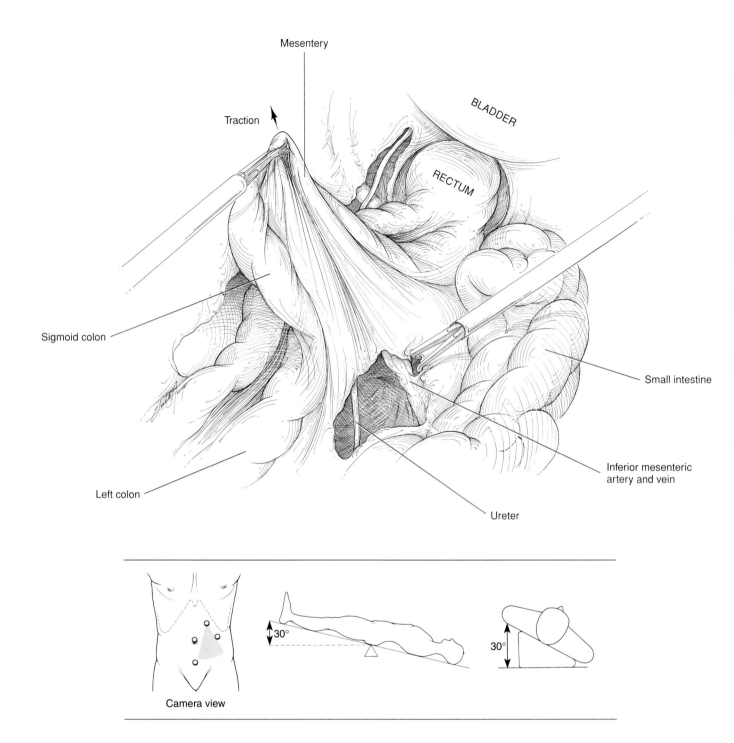

Mesentery

Traction

BLADDER

RECTUM

Sigmoid colon

Small intestine

Inferior mesenteric
artery and vein

Left colon

Ureter

Camera view

30°

30°

E   A Babcock clamp inserted through the umbilical trocar is used to apply superior traction to the mesentery. The peritoneum at the base of the vessels is incised and the inferior mesenteric vessels are separated.

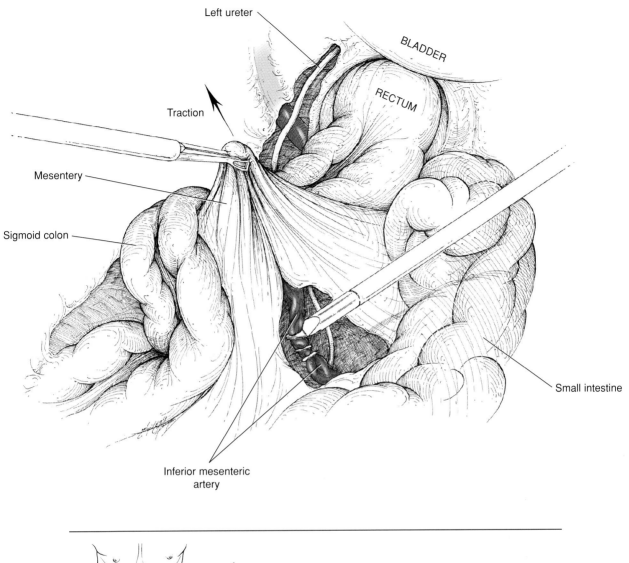

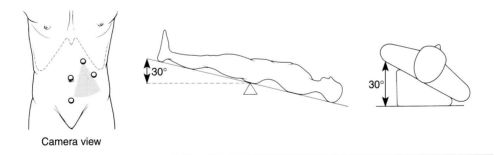

F   The mesenteric vessels are individually ligated with a clip applier inserted through the suprapubic trocar.

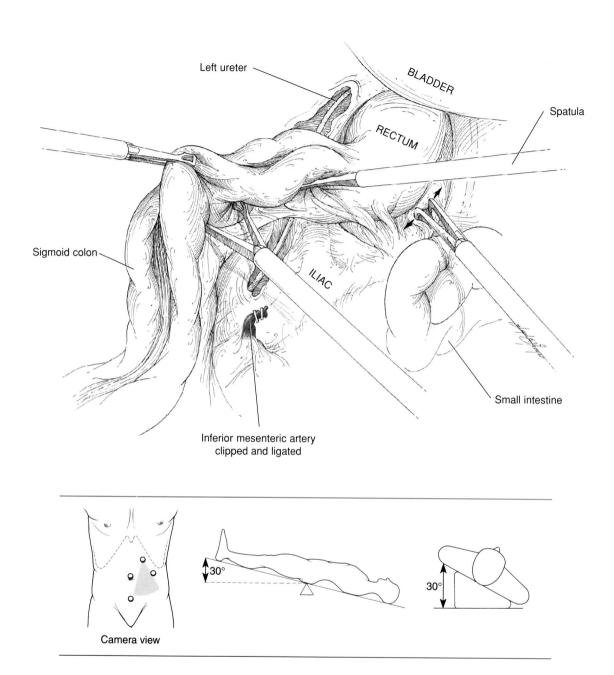

Left ureter

BLADDER

RECTUM

Spatula

Sigmoid colon

ILIAC

Small intestine

Inferior mesenteric artery
clipped and ligated

Camera view

30°

30°

G   The entire course of the left ureter is exposed.

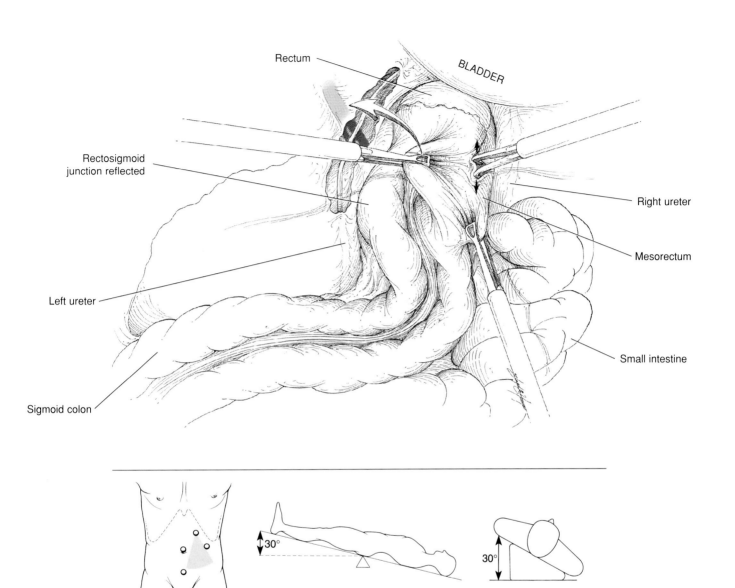

Rectum

BLADDER

Rectosigmoid
junction reflected

Right ureter

Mesorectum

Left ureter

Small intestine

Sigmoid colon

30°

30°

Camera view

H   The lateral stalks are easily identified and developed by the surgeon
with a right-angle clamp inserted through the suprapubic trocar. The
assistant applies traction to the rectum superiorly and laterally and
countertraction is directed medially via the umbilical trocar.

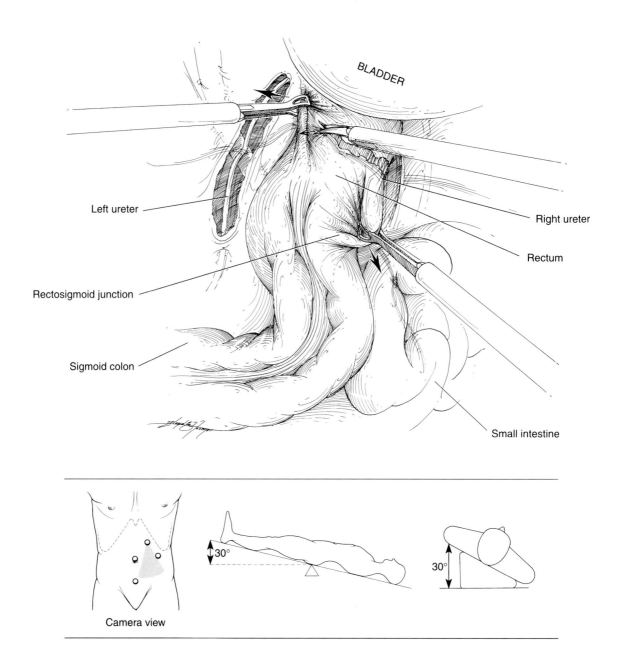

BLADDER

Left ureter

Right ureter

Rectum

Rectosigmoid junction

Sigmoid colon

Small intestine

Camera view

30°

30°

I   The anterior rectovesicular peritoneal investiture is sharply incised with cautery scissors through the suprapubic trocar.

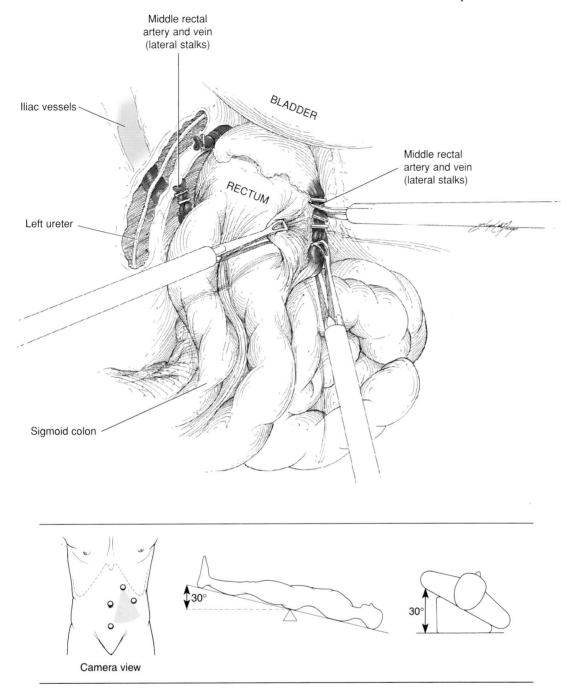

Middle rectal
artery and vein
(lateral stalks)

Iliac vessels

BLADDER

Middle rectal
artery and vein
(lateral stalks)

RECTUM

Left ureter

Sigmoid colon

Camera view

30°

30°

J   Lateral stalks are clipped and transected. Clips and cautery scissors are
applied through the suprapubic trocar.

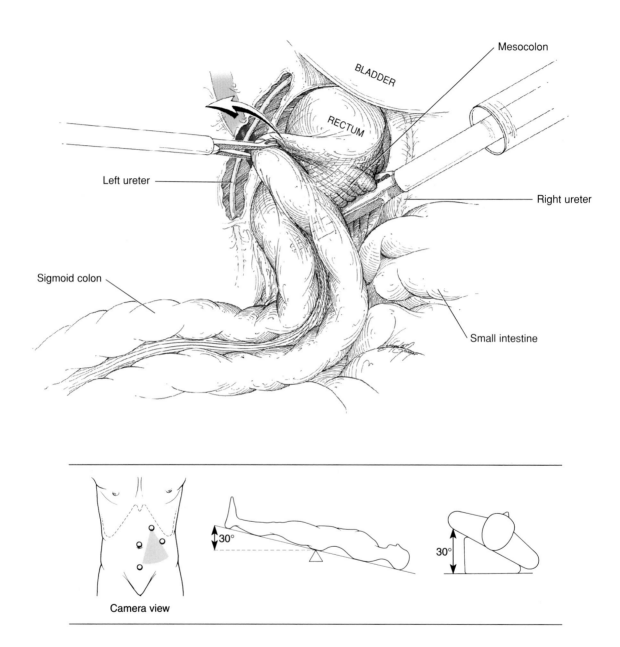

K   The mesorectum is with a stapling device.

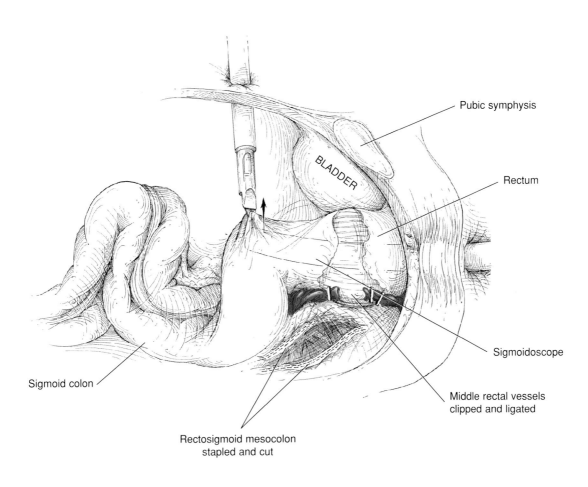

Pubic symphysis

BLADDER

Rectum

Sigmoidoscope

Middle rectal vessels
clipped and ligated

Sigmoid colon

Rectosigmoid mesocolon
stapled and cut

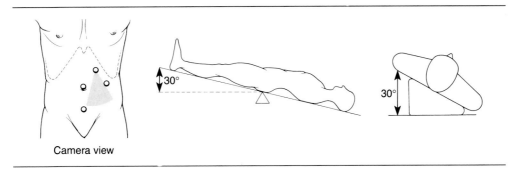

Camera view

30°

30°

L The devascularization of the mesorectum is shown after application of
the endolinear stapler.

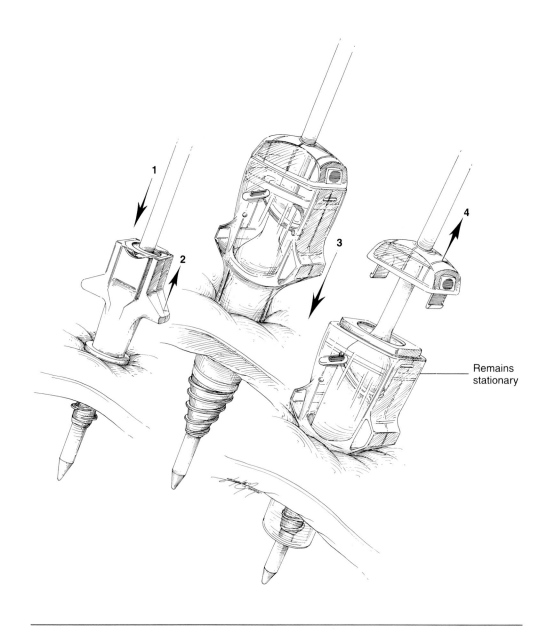

M Conversion of the suprapubic trocar to an 18 mm trocar. Step 1, a guidebar is inserted into the existing trocar. Step 2, the 12 mm trocar is removed, leaving the guidebar. Step 3, after extending the skin incision, the 18 mm trocar is inserted over the guidebar. Step 4, the guidebar and insert are removed, leaving the 18 mm trocar.

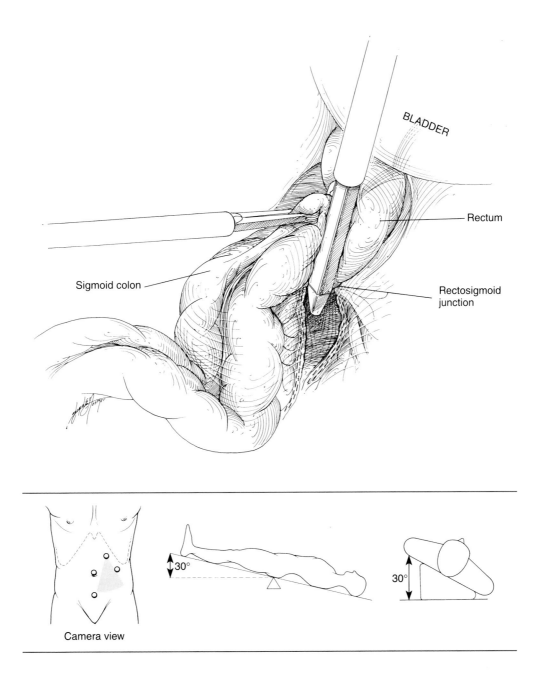

N   The endolinear stapler is positioned at the proximal margin of the mobilized rectum. This stapler is inserted through the suprapubic 18 mm
trocar.

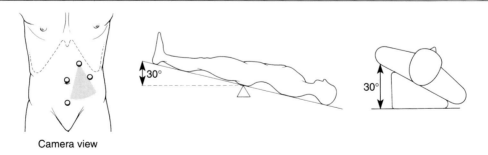

O   Transection of the sigmoid colon in preparation for colostomy.

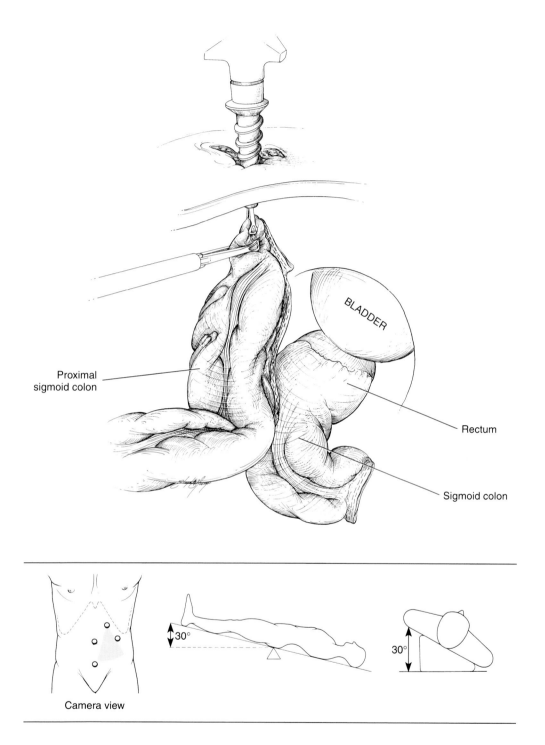

Proximal
sigmoid colon

BLADDER

Rectum

Sigmoid colon

Camera view

30°

30°

P   Delivery of the proximal bowel through the incision in the anterior
abdominal wall.

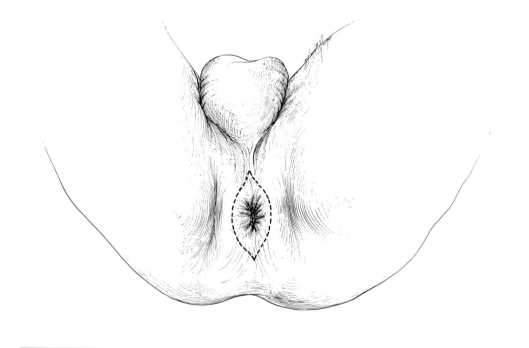

Q   A traditional circumanal perineal incision.

10

Total Abdominal Colectomy

W. Peter Geis ▪ Gustavo Plasencia ▪ Moises Jacobs ▪
Philip F. Caushaj

General Considerations

The total abdominal colectomy is the most challenging procedure performed laparoscopically. It incorporates a right colectomy, left colectomy, and sigmoid resection with the inherent technical challenges of all three procedures. The two flexures, hepatic and splenic, require mobilization. The ureters require identification. This procedure should only be attempted by an experienced laparoscopic surgeon. Abdominal colectomy is indicated for multiple polyps that are endoscopically irremovable, familial polyposis syndromes, multiple polyposis syndromes, colonic inertia, inflammatory bowel disease, multiple neoplasms of the colon, and ischemic colitis.

Preoperative Setup and Trocar Placement

The operating room setup and trocar placement are as shown in Fig. *A*. Two video monitors are positioned to the left and right of the patient. The patient is placed in a modified lithotomy position. The surgeon stands to the right of the patient, while the assistant is either between the patient's legs or to the lower right of the patient. Four 10/12 mm trocars are required. The first trocar is inserted into the umbilicus, and a diagnostic laparoscopy is performed. If there is no contraindication to the laparoscopic technique, the additional 10/12 mm trocars are opened and inserted under direct vision. The secondary trocars are placed in the right and left suprapubic areas and the epigastrium.

Mobilization and Devascularization
LEFT COLON

Left colonic mobilization is attempted first because it is the more technically challenging part of the operation. If technical difficulties occur, less time will have been spent on the laparoscopic portion of the operation.

The assistant relocates the video camera to the right suprapubic trocar. The operating room table is placed in reverse Trendelenburg position with a right oblique rotation (with a minimal elevation of 30 degrees). The monitor on the patient's left is at the patient's feet. This monitor will be moved toward the head of the table as the dissection proceeds toward the splenic flexure. Fig. *B* shows the critical components of left colon mobilization. The assistant directs the video camera through the right suprapubic trocar while a Babcock clamp in the left suprapubic trocar applies medial traction to the left colon. The surgeon incises the peritoneal attachments of the left colon with cautery scissors that have been placed through the umbilical trocar and applies traction to the descending colon with a Babcock clamp in the epigastric trocar.

Once the peritoneal attachments of the sigmoid and descending colon are sharply incised, the left colon is reflected medially. After the left ureter is identified, the left ureter and the descending and sigmoid colon are mobilized medially, then the splenic flexure is mobilized. The video camera remains in the right suprapubic trocar; however, we prefer a 30-degree laparoscope for this part of the operation. The assistant applies medial traction to the descending colon with a Babcock clamp in the left suprapubic trocar, while the surgeon retracts the distal transverse colon inferiorly and medially with a Babcock clamp in the epigastric trocar. Takedown of the splenic flexure requires division of the phrenocolic, splenocolic, and renocolic ligaments. These are incised by the surgeon with cautery scissors through the umbilical trocar, working from the television monitor to the upper left of the patient.

Once the splenic flexure is mobilized, the surgeon must decide whether to remove the greater omentum. If it is not to be removed, dissection continues in the avascular plane between the greater omentum and transverse colon. The video camera remains in the right suprapubic trocar. Traction to the transverse colon is applied inferiorly by the assistant with a Babcock clamp through the left suprapubic port. Countertraction to the greater omentum is delivered by the surgeon with a Babcock clamp in the epigastric trocar. Dissection in this avascular plane is performed with cautery scissors through the umbilical trocar to the level of the proximal transverse colon.

If the greater omentum is to be removed en bloc with the colon, traction to the transverse colon remains the same; however, the surgeon should apply countertraction to the superior edge of the gastrocolic ligament. This ligament is vascular and should be divided between clips. The dissection should proceed to the level of the midtransverse colon.

The surgeon must decide whether intracorporeal devascularization is required. If no intracorporeal devascularization is necessary, the surgeon proceeds to right colon and hepatic flexure mobilization. However, we will describe our technique for intracorporeal devascularization. Since the entire left colon and distal transverse colon have been mobilized at this juncture, the blood supply is now approached. The video camera remains in the right suprapubic trocar. The descending colon and sigmoid colon mesentery are placed under tension by Babcock clamps inserted through the epigastric and left suprapubic trocar, which are held by the surgeon and assistant, respectively. The surgeon incises the peritoneal surface of the mesentery with cautery scissors applied through the umbilical trocar. Precautions must be taken to avoid injury of the ureter. Once the inferior mesenteric vessels have been identified, separated, and ligated, the remainder of the mesentery is divided between clips to the level of the sacral promontory. After reexamining the location of the left ureter, devascularization proceeds proximally to the left branch of the middle colic artery.

RIGHT COLON

Mobilization and devascularization of the right colon is now performed. The surgeon is positioned to the left of the patient and the assistant remains between the patient's legs. The patient is placed in Trendelenburg position with a left lateral oblique rotation. The camera is relocated to the left suprapubic trocar. Medial traction to the cecum is applied by a Babcock clamp in the right suprapubic trocar. The ascending colon is retracted medially by the surgeon with a Babcock clamp in the umbilical trocar. Cautery scissors, placed in the epigastric trocar, are used to incise the peritoneal investiture from the terminal ileum to the hepatic flexure.

After the right colon is mobilized, the position of the patient and instruments changes once again. The patient is placed in reverse Trendelenburg position. The video camera remains in the left suprapubic trocar. Traction is applied to the distal ascending colon by a Babcock clamp in the right suprapubic trocar, while the surgeon applies inferior countertraction to the hepatic flexure directly with a Babcock clamp in the umbilical trocar. Division of the hepatocolic ligament is accomplished by the use of either cautery scissors or clips placed through the epigastric trocar. The duodenum is identified and the developmental adhesions between the duodenum and mesentery are divided. If indicated, the ureter should be identified now.

The right transverse colon is mobilized to meet the dissection carried out on the left. The video camera remains in the left suprapubic trocar. Inferior traction to the proximal transverse colon is directed by the assistant with a Babcock clamp through the right suprapubic trocar. The greater omentum is reflected anteriorly by the surgeon with a Babcock clamp inserted in the epigastric trocar. Cautery scissors directed through the umbilical trocar are used to dissect in the avascular plane between the greater omentum and transverse colon. As mentioned previously, if the greater omentum is to be removed, the setup remains the same, except the surgeon exerts anterior traction to the superior edge of the gastrocolic ligament. The ligament is transected between hemoclips. At this juncture, the mobilizations of the entire abdominal colon are complete.

If intracorporeal devascularization has been performed on the left, we proceed with intracorporeal devascularization on the right. The video camera remains in the left suprapubic trocar. Tension is applied to the mesentery of the right colon with Babcock clamps inserted through the epigastric and right suprapubic trocars by the surgeon and assistant, respectively. The blood supply is ligated as described in Chapter 7. Nevertheless, the surgeon scores the mesentery with cautery scissors placed through the umbilical trocar. The vessels are developed and divided between clips. Alternatively, these vessels may be divided with a vascular endolinear cutter. Once the ileocolic vessels have been divided, a mesenteric window, as previously described, becomes evident. The right colic and middle colic vessels are then sequentially clipped and ligated. This completes the intracorporeal devascularization.

Resection and Extracorporeal Anastomosis

The conduct of the remainder of the operation depends on whether an intracorporeal or extracorporeal anastomosis is performed and what type of procedure is planned. In this section we will review extracorporeal anastomosis and resection. The options are to perform a total abdominal colectomy with ileorectal anastomosis, an ileal pouch anal anastomosis, or an abdominal colectomy with an end ileostomy and a Hartmann's pouch.

After the colon has been mobilized and intracorporeal devascularization accomplished, a Pfannenstiel incision is made. This incision may incorporate the right and left suprapubic trocar sites. The specimen is delivered through the incision and a standard resection carried out. The ileorectal anastomosis and/or end ileostomy and Hartmann's pouch are created under direct vision. If an ileal pouch anal anastomosis is to be performed, then mobilization of the rectum proceeds, through the Pfannenstiel incision, as for an open procedure. Once the abdominal colon and rectum have been resected at the level of the anal canal, a standard pouch that has been created from the ileum is fashioned and double-stapled to the anus. A protective loop ileostomy is brought up through a previously marked site. An alternative procedure is a complete intracorporeal ileoanal anastomotic procedure; this is technically challenging.

Resection and Intracorporeal Anastomosis

Resection may be accomplished intracorporeally. After mobilization and devascularization of the abdominal colon, the terminal ileum is transected with an endolinear stapling device inserted through the epigastric trocar. The specimen is then delivered through a small assisting incision in the left lower quadrant or delivered through the rectum. We avoid removing the specimen through the anorectal sphincter mechanism because of concerns that have been expressed in the literature regarding transient and/or permanent injury to the anorectal sphincter complex.

Intracorporeal anastomosis is then accomplished, depending on the operation. The options are ileorectal anastomosis, an ileoanal pouch anastomotic procedure, or creation of a Hartmann's pouch and end ileostomy. The technique for ileorectal anastomosis is similar to that for low anterior resection (see Chapter 8).

Proctocolectomy

Mobilization and devascularization of the abdominal colon have been accomplished as just described. The operating room setup changes once again. The patient is placed in steep Trendelenburg position, rotated to the right lateral oblique. The video camera is positioned in the epigastric trocar. Traction is applied to the sigmoid colon laterally and anteriorly by a Babcock clamp directed by the assistant through the right suprapubic trocar. The surgeon lifts the rectosigmoid anteriorly with a Babcock clamp inserted in the umbilical trocar. Cautery scissors or a spatula is inserted through the left suprapubic trocar and the retrorectal space is entered. The monitors are at the patient's feet.

The retrorectal space is mobilized to the level of the levator ani muscles after Waldeyer's fascia is incised. Then the rectovesicular peritoneal investiture is incised, and the remainder of the operation proceeds as described in Chapter 11. After removal of the specimen, an ileostomy is delivered through a previously marked stoma site in the left lower quadrant.

Clinical Caveats

- The left colon mobilization and takedown of the splenic flexure should be performed first. If technical difficulties are encountered and conversion to an open procedure is necessary, this will be evident be carried out early in the procedure.

- Multiple monitors are required on both sides of the patient, and these may need to be relocated during the procedure. Positioning for the scrub nurse and instrument tray must be fluid because of the dynamic nature of this procedure.

- If the procedure is performed for malignancy, the greater omentum is removed en bloc.

- When ligating the middle colic vessels, anatomic certainty is crucial to avoid ligation of celiac vessels or superior mesenteric vessels.

Surgical Technique

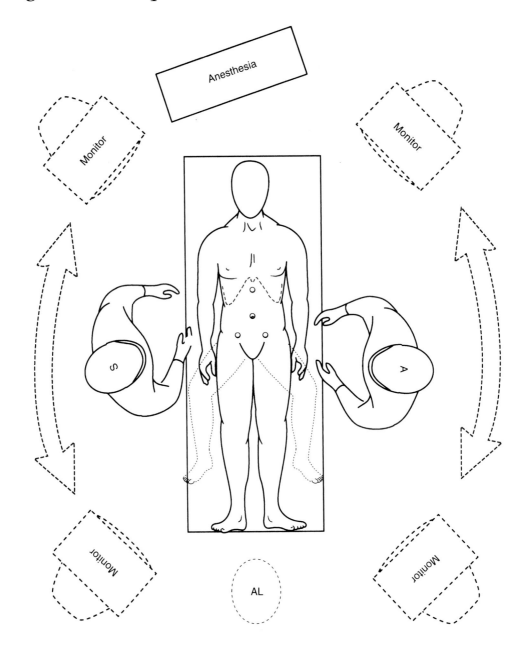

A Operating room setup for total abdominal colectomy. The positions of the surgeon, assistant, and TV monitors are variable (see text). *S,* surgeon; *A,* assistant; *AL,* alternative position for assistant. Note suggested trocar placement.

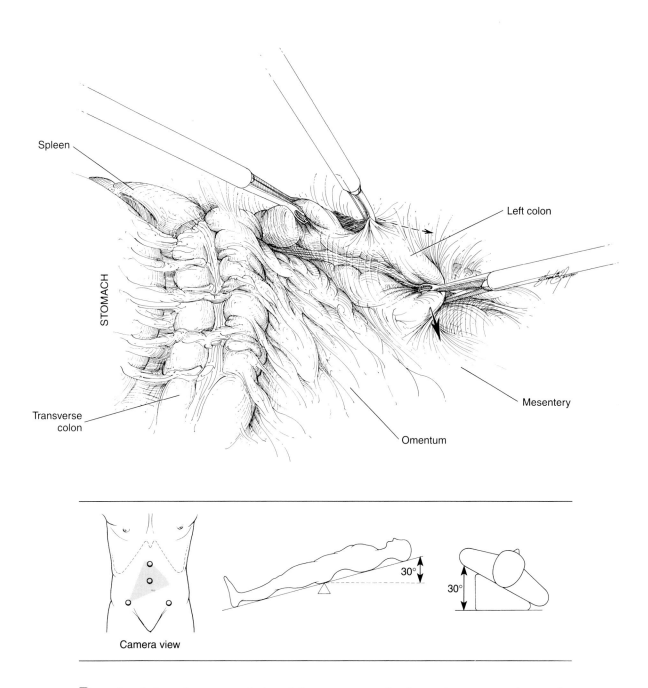

B   The left colon is mobilized by incising the lateral peritoneal attachments.

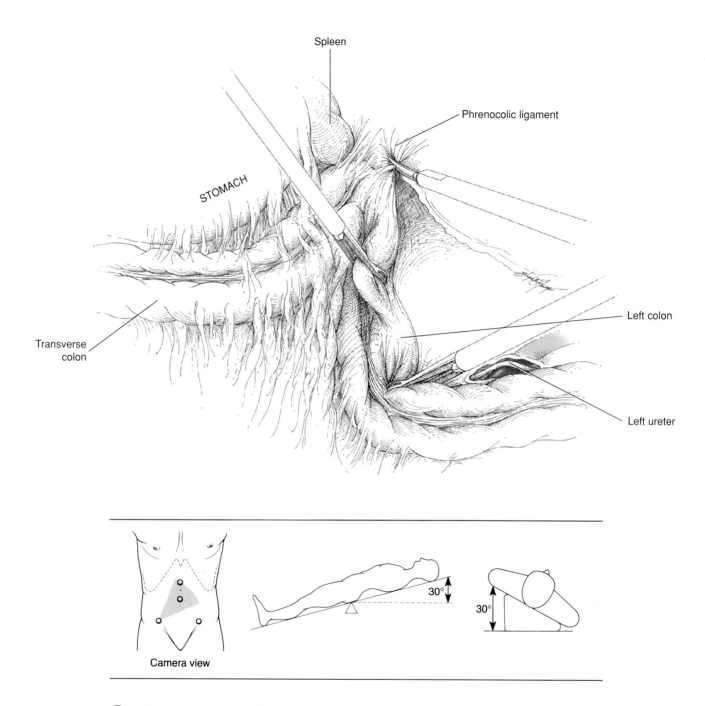

Spleen

Phrenocolic ligament

STOMACH

Transverse colon

Left colon

Left ureter

Camera view

30°

30°

C The takedown of the splenic flexure is performed by incising the splenocolic and phrenocolic ligaments.

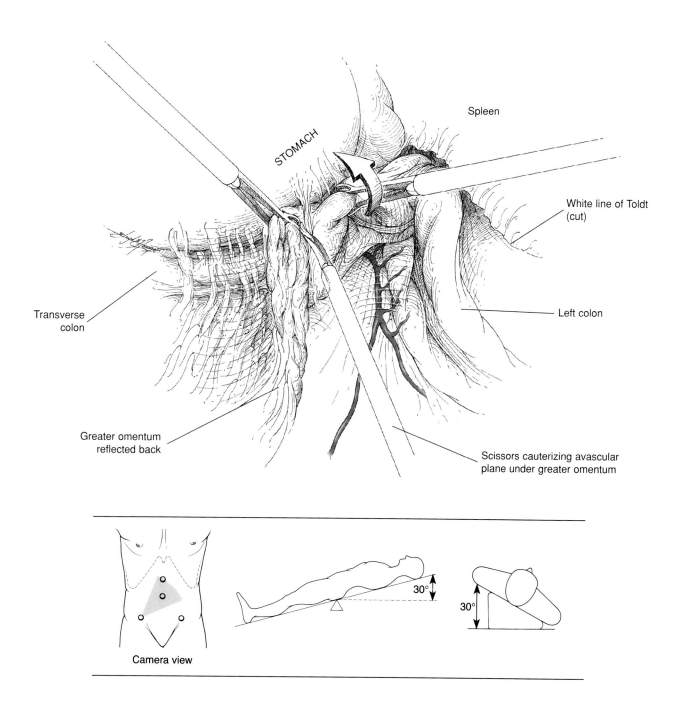

Spleen

STOMACH

White line of Toldt
(cut)

Left colon

Transverse
colon

Greater omentum
reflected back

Scissors cauterizing avascular
plane under greater omentum

Camera view

30°

30°

D   Superior traction is applied to the distal transverse colon while transecting the gastrocolic ligament.

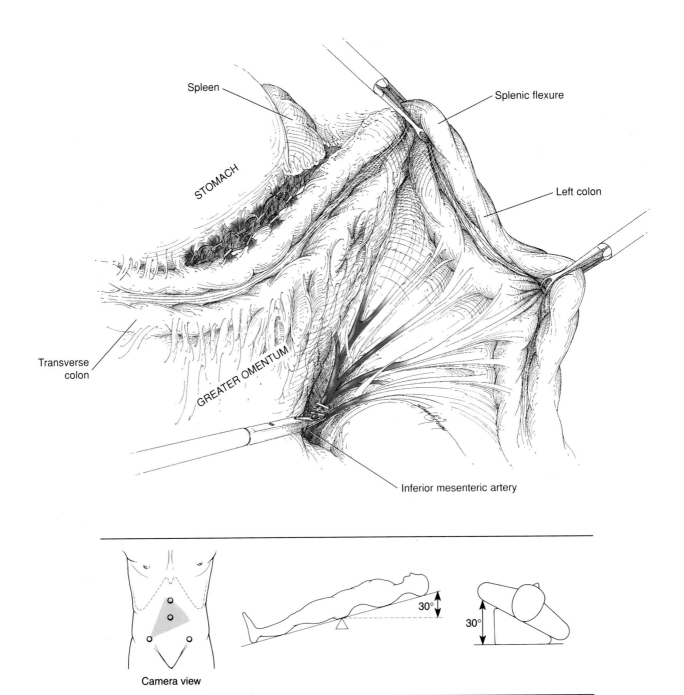

E Traction is applied laterally to the mobilized colon. These forces of traction cause vessels to bow while the left colic vessels are ligated.

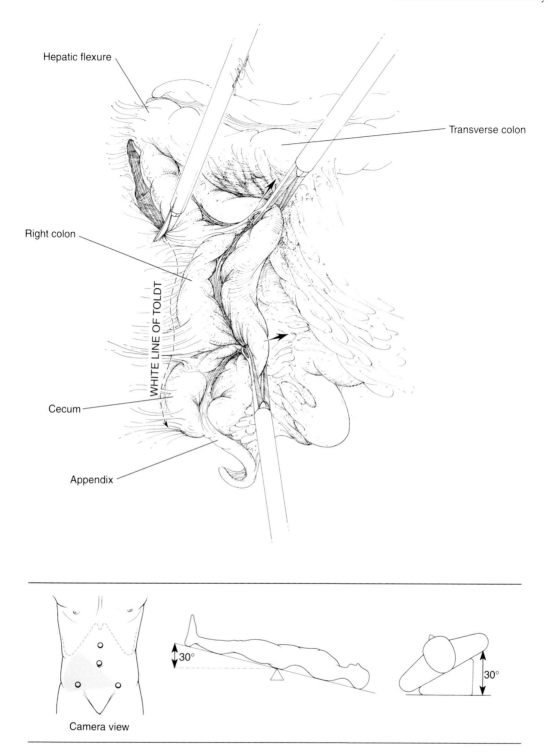

Hepatic flexure

Transverse colon

Right colon

WHITE LINE OF TOLDT

Cecum

Appendix

Camera view

30°

30°

F   The peritoneal attachments of the right colon are mobilized. The patient is moved to the Trendelenburg position, left lateral oblique. The camera is relocated to the left suprapubic port.

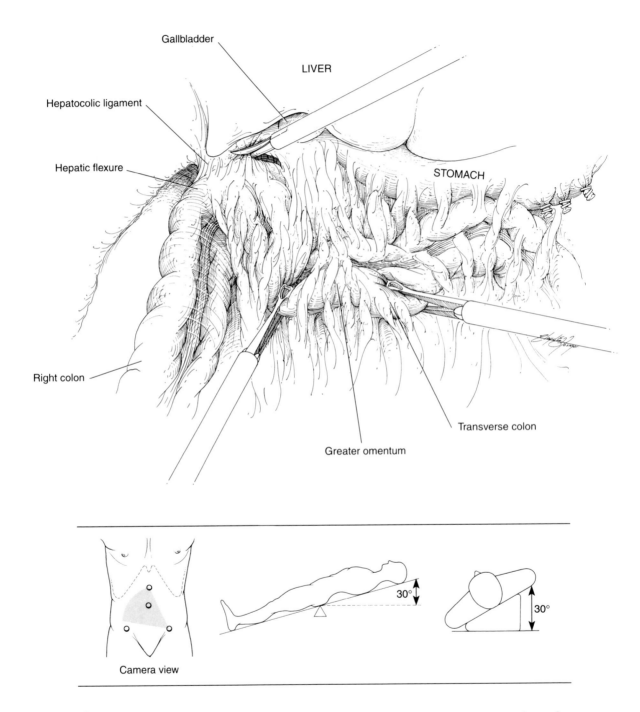

Gallbladder

LIVER

Hepatocolic ligament

Hepatic flexure

STOMACH

Right colon

Transverse colon

Greater omentum

30°

30°

Camera view

G   For the takedown of the hepatic flexure, the patient is moved to the reverse Trendelenburg position.

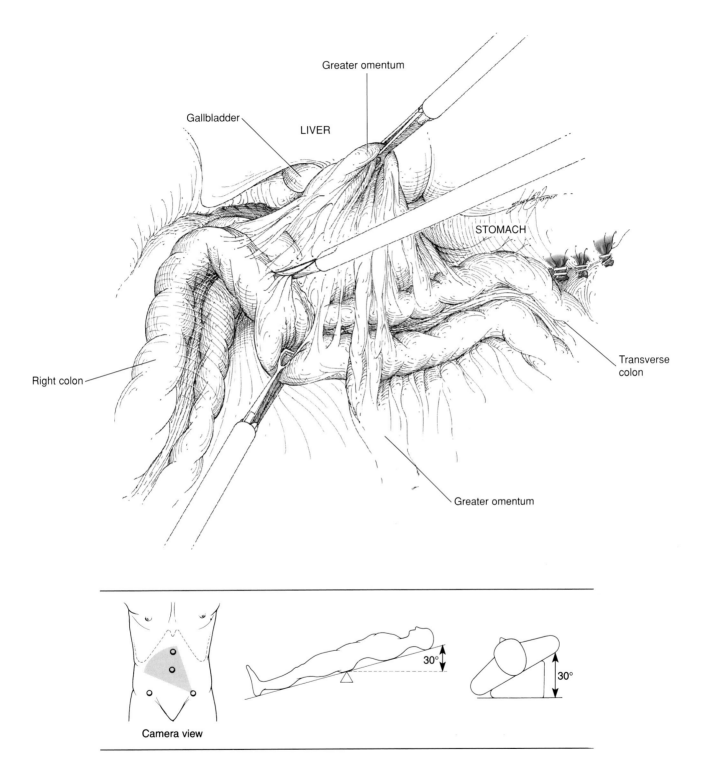

H Dissection of the greater omentum from the transverse colon.

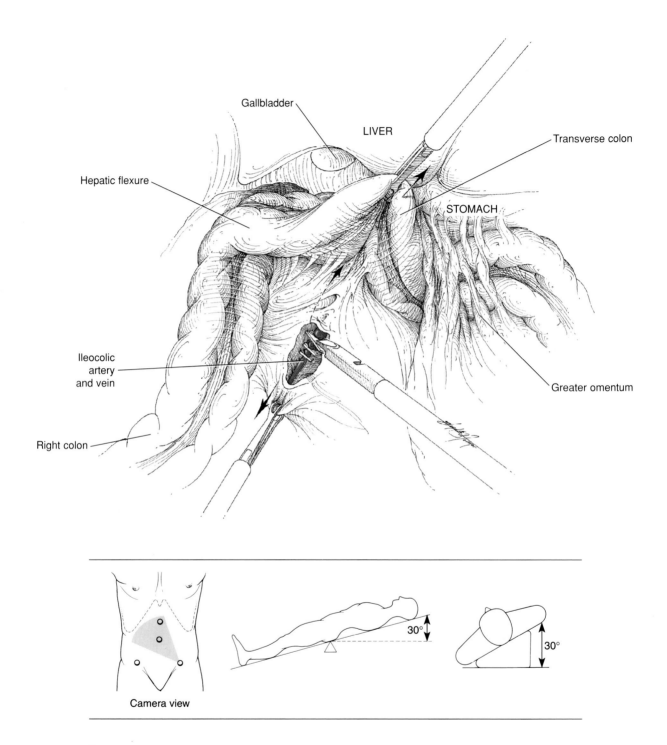

Gallbladder

LIVER

Transverse colon

Hepatic flexure

STOMACH

Ileocolic
artery
and vein

Greater omentum

Right colon

30°

30°

Camera view

I Ligation of the ileocolic vessel is facilitated by traction superiorly to the transverse colon and inferiorly to the mesentery.

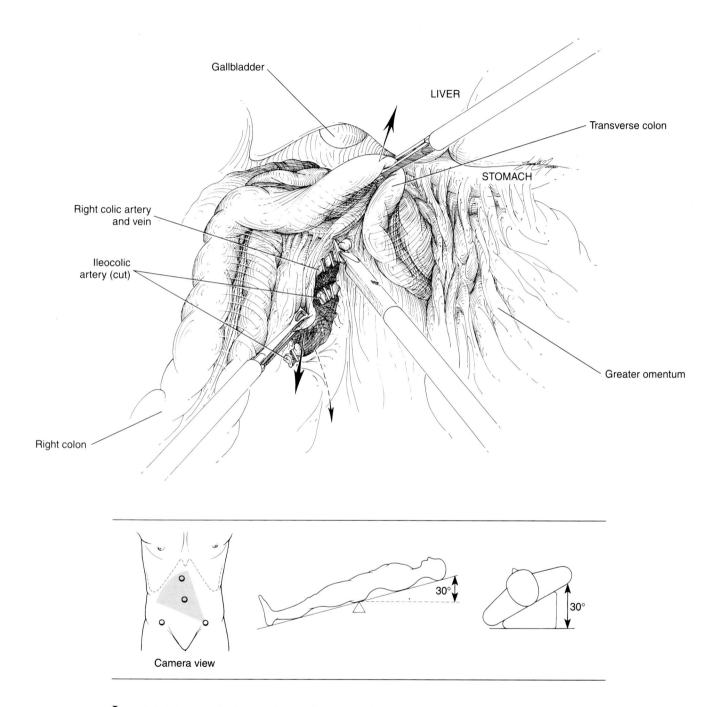

J Division of the right colic vessels. It is essential to determine the anatomic locations of the vessels before ligation to avoid iatrogenic injury to the superior mesenteric vessels.

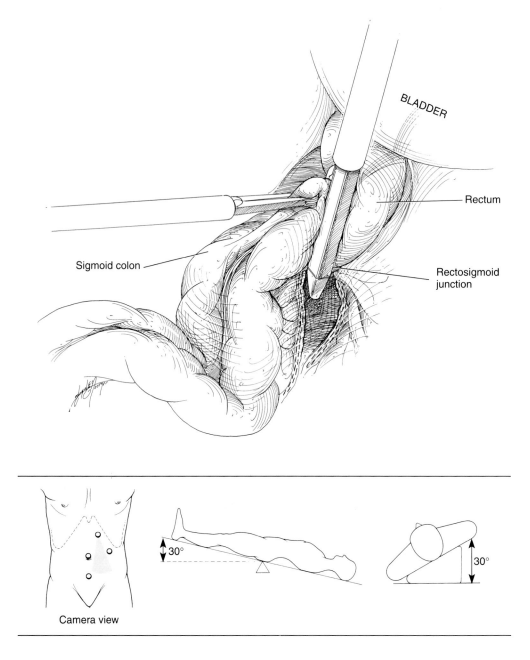

K   The patient is repositioned to the Trendelenburg position, left lateral oblique, and the camera is moved to the epigastric port. The stapling device is positioned at the distal anastomotic site.

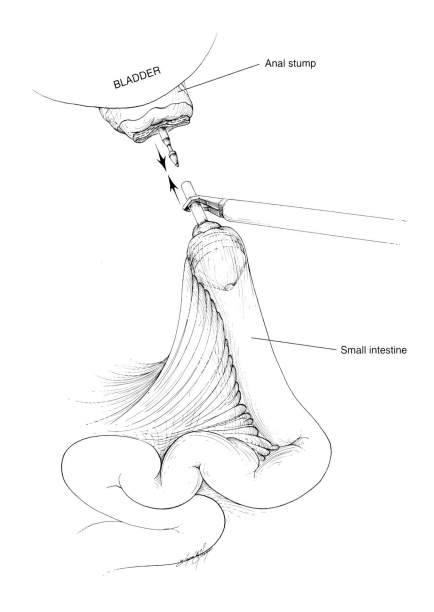

L   OPTION 1: Following resection, extraction of the specimen, and insertion of the anvil into the proximal colon (see Chapter 7), the ileorectal anastomosis is completed.

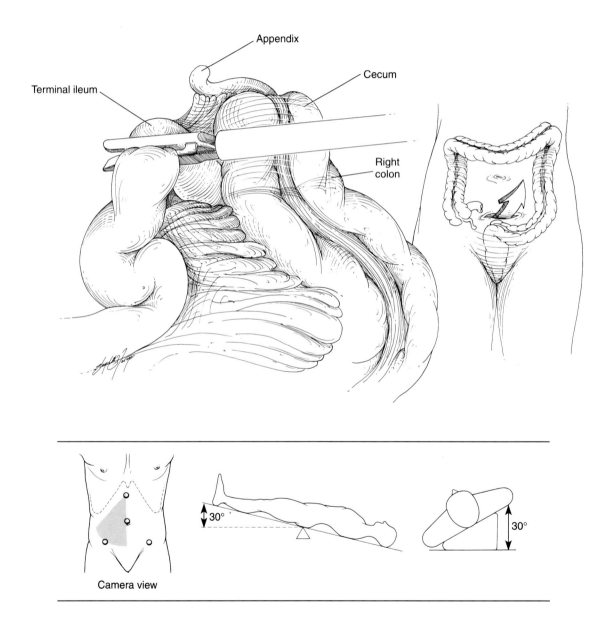

M OPTION 2: Transection of the terminal ileum in preparation for J pouch. The patient may be positioned in the left lateral oblique rotation during J pouch preparation.

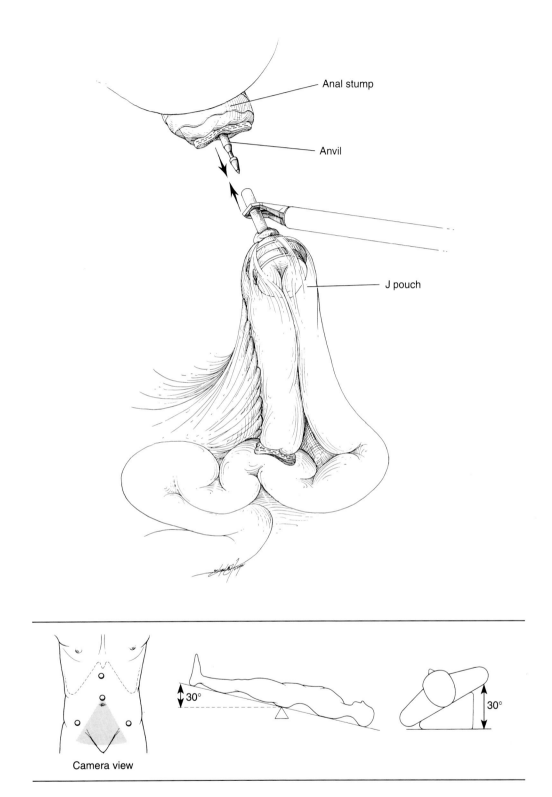

N OPTION 2, cont'd: Anastomosis of the J pouch to the anus.

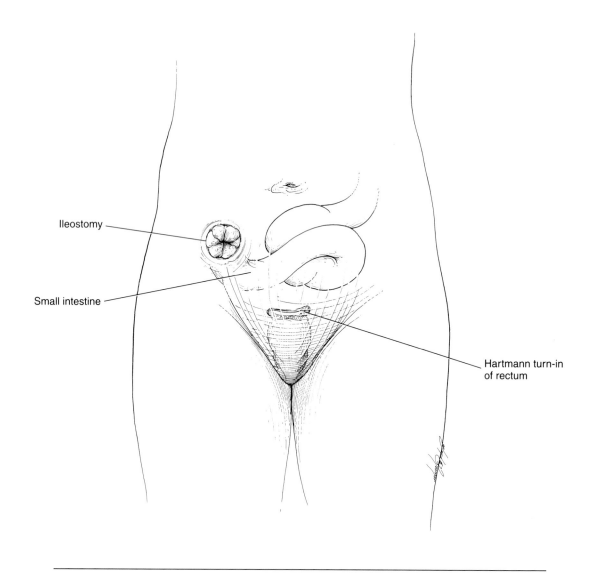

Ileostomy

Small intestine

Hartmann turn-in
of rectum

O   OPTION 3: Creation of end ileostomy and Hartmann turn-in of the rectum following a total abdominal colectomy.

11

Colostomy Formation and Closure

Moises Jacobs ▪ Gustavo Plasencia ▪ Philip F. Caushaj

General Considerations

The creation and closure of colostomy may turn out to be the procedure of choice for the laparoscopic technique. The indications for creation of colostomy are the same for laparoscopic procedures as for open procedures. The takedown and closure of a Hartmann turn-in and colostomy are the primary indications for the initial surgery. The Hartmann closure will be laparoscopically feasible, depending on the nature of the patient's pelvis. If there are numerous adhesions and small bowel matted to the pelvis, these closures may not be indicated.

Colostomy Formation
PREOPERATIVE SETUP AND TROCAR PLACEMENT

Preoperatively the patient is evaluated by an enterostomal therapist and the colostomy site is marked on the abdomen. The preoperative setup of the operating room and trocar placement is shown in Fig. *A*. Two television monitors are positioned at either side of the patient's feet. The surgeon is positioned to the right of the patient, while the assistant is to the left. The patient is placed in a modified lithotomy position.

The first 10/12 mm trocar is inserted through the umbilicus, and a diagnostic laparoscopy is performed before secondary trocars are placed. If there is no contraindication to laparoscopy, the secondary trocars are placed: in the left midclavicular line; approximately two fingerbreadths below the left costal margin; and suprapubically. If a fourth trocar is required, it is placed laterally in the anterior axillary line (left flank) at the level of the umbilicus.

MOBILIZATION

The laparoscope is placed in the left upper quadrant trocar. The surgeon applies medial traction to the sigmoid colon with a Babcock clamp through the umbilical trocar, while cautery scissors in the suprapubic trocar are employed to sharply incise the peritoneal attachments of the sigmoid colon. Since no devascularization is performed, we do not routinely identify the ureter.

After the sigmoid and descending colon are fully mobilized, the surgeon must decide whether to create an end colostomy or loop colostomy. If a loop colostomy is to be formed, the previously marked stoma site is incised and the stoma fashioned. A Babcock clamp is inserted through the suprapubic trocar and delivers the sigmoid to the anterior abdominal wall at the stoma site (Fig. *C*). The stoma site is then opened through all layers, including posterior fascia and peritoneum. This causes immediate loss of the pneumoperitoneum. The Babcock clamp in the suprapubic trocar delivers the mobilized colon through the incision. This technique minimizes the time necessary to deliver the sigmoid colon and also reduces the possibility of bowel torsion.

Once the sigmoid is exteriorized, a standard loop colostomy is created. A pneumoperitoneum is reestablished, and the colon is evaluated for torsion and hemostasis. Secondary trocars are removed under direct vision and all incisions are closed.

If an end colostomy is indicated, the left ureter must be identified as described earlier. The sigmoid colon is retracted medially with a Babcock clamp in the umbilical trocar, while the surgeon dissects and identifies the ureter using a right-angle clamp through the suprapubic trocar. Once the ureter is identified, the bowel is divided at a position that easily reaches the anterior abdominal wall with a 35 mm endolinear stapling device placed through the suprapubic trocar. Occasionally two firings may be required to divide the bowel; however, this is the exception. When transecting the bowel with the endolinear cutter, traction is applied to the bowel with a Babcock clamp inserted through the umbilical trocar. The mesentery should also be divided to enable the proximal colon to be delivered through the anterior abdominal wall at the stoma site. Fig. 11-1 depicts division of the mesentery using a vascular endolinear stapling device. The reach of the proximal colon to the anterior abdominal wall at the colostomy site is tested. If the proximal colon reaches the abdominal wall without tension, an incision is made at the colostomy site. The proximal colon is delivered

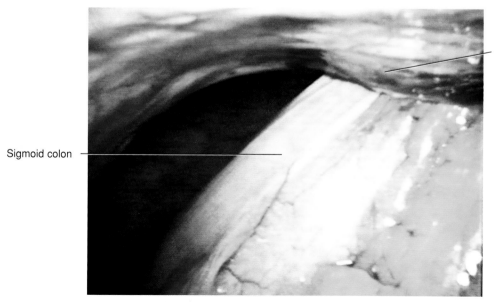

Fig. 11-1. Exteriorization of the colon with no tension.

through the stoma site by a Babcock clamp inserted through the suprapubic trocar. Once it is externalized, a standard colostomy is fashioned.

Although the examples mentioned are for end or loop sigmoid colostomy, the same principles can be applied to any segment of the colon or small bowel, in particular transverse colostomy or ileostomy. Mobilization of the desired segment of bowel to reach the anterior abdominal wall without tension and transection of the bowel or mesentery is necessary to create an end stoma.

Colostomy Closure
PREOPERATIVE SETUP AND TROCAR PLACEMENT

Unlike the setup for sigmoid resection or low anterior resection, the operating room is configured differently for colostomy closure. Two television monitors are necessary, both to the left of the patient—one at the foot of the operating table and the other at the head of the table. The television monitor must be placed at the head of the table because of the frequent need for takedown of the splenic flexure. Unlike the previously described laparoscopic procedures, we do not create a pneumoperitoneum and perform laparoscopy at this juncture.

MOBILIZATION

Before proceeding with pneumoperitoneum and laparoscopy, the colostomy site is freed from the mucocutaneous juncture, subcutaneous tissue, and the fascial adhesions (Fig. 11-2). The abdominal cavity is entered and any soft adhesions surrounding the intraperitoneal colostomy site are bluntly dissected. A purse-string suture is applied to the colostomy site, and the head and anvil of the circular stapling device is placed into the bowel (Figs. 11-3 and 11-4). The purse-string is secured, leaving the tails of the suture long, and the colon and the head and anvil are returned to the abdominal cavity. Pneumoperitoneum is established by placing a trocar into the colostomy site. The skin and fascia may need to be secured to maintain a seal with towel clips. The video camera is placed through this left lower quadrant trocar, and diagnostic laparoscopy is performed. If intraperitoneal adhesions are minimal, a second trocar may be placed in the midline between the umbilicus and the suprapubic line.

The rectal stump can be identified by placing the shaft of the circular stapler transanally and displacing the rectum anteriorly. If no small bowel is adherent in the pelvis and the anterior rectal wall is free, the spearhead can be extruded through the anterior rectal wall. The surgeon can direct union of the head and anvil with the spearhead with a specially designed grasper directed through the midline trocar. Using this technique, if no ex-

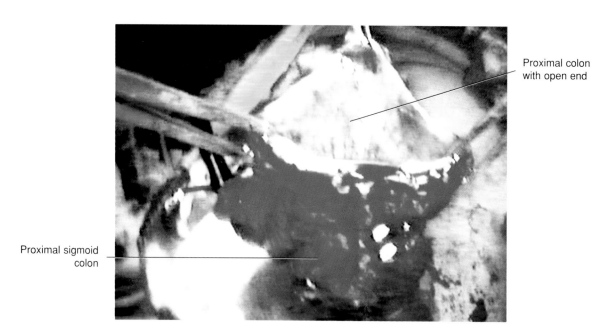

Proximal colon
with open end

Proximal sigmoid
colon

Fig. 11-2. Opening of the proximal colon for placement of the head and anvil of the circular stapler.

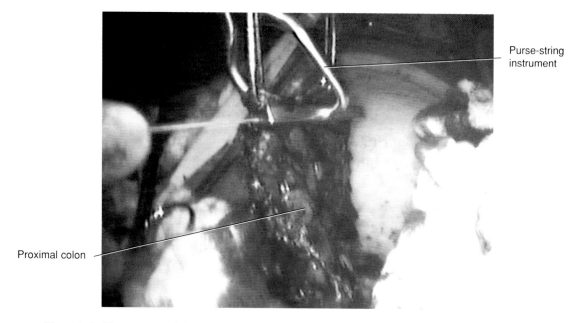

Purse-string
instrument

Proximal colon

Fig. 11-3. Placement of the purse-string instrument on the proximal sigmoid colon for passage of the head and anvil of the circular stapler.

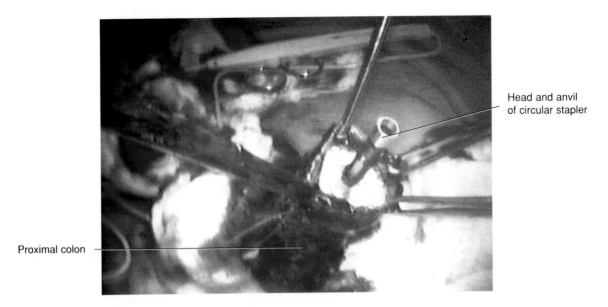

Head and anvil
of circular stapler

Proximal colon

Fig. 11-4. Placement of the head and anvil of the circular stapler in the proximal colon.

tensive enterolysis or small bowel mobilization is required, it is possible to close a Hartmann's pouch with the use of only two trocars.

If there are significant adhesions surrounding the intraperitoneal colostomy site that preclude adequate visualization of the peritoneal cavity when the video camera is inserted through the colostomy site trocar, we select a remote site to place the second trocar. This is one of the few situations in which we routinely employ the Hasson open technique. The site most frequently used is the right upper quadrant. After the second trocar has been inserted and pneumoperitoneum established, the video camera is relocated to this trocar. If intraperitoneal adhesions are not extensive, at which point we would convert to an open procedure, a third trocar is placed under direct vision into the right lower quadrant. The surgeon uses cautery scissors or a dissecting instrument through this right lower quadrant trocar to free the intraperitoneal adhesions, predominantly around the colostomy site, the midline adhesion, and pelvis.

ANASTOMOSIS

If the adhesions around the colostomy site can be freed, then the video camera is once again relocated to the left lower quadrant trocar. The assistant moves to the left of the patient, while the surgeon continues the procedure with instruments inserted in the right upper and lower quadrant trocars. The right upper quadrant is used to place a Babcock clamp to apply traction while the right lower quadrant trocar directs the cautery scissors or dissecting instrument.

After dissection has freed up the intraperitoneal adhesions, the surgeon analyzes the degree of tension between the proximal colon and the rectum. If the level of tension is significant, then the surgeon will take down the splenic flexure. Viewing the television monitor at the patient's head, with the video camera directed through the left lower quadrant trocar, the surgeon applies medial traction to the splenic flexure with a Babcock clamp through the right upper quadrant trocar, then frees the ligamentous attachments of the splenic flexure with cautery scissors through the right lower quadrant trocar. The splenic flexure mobilization follows the same principles discussed in previous chapters.

After takedown of the splenic flexure is accomplished, the operating team views the television monitor at the foot of the operating room table. The proximal colon, with head and anvil, is now joined to the extruded spearhead using the previously described technique. The circular stapling device is fired. After removing the stapling device, the doughnuts of bowel are inspected for structural integrity. The anastomosis is tested by inflating the rectum with air administered via a proctoscope inserted transanally. If anastomotic integrity is documented, the abdomen is examined for hemostasis and the secondary trocars are removed under direct vision. The incisions are closed.

Clinical Caveats

- The patient who is being considered for creation of a stoma should be evaluated preoperatively by an enterostomal therapist for proper stoma site location.

- When creating a stoma, there is no vascular ligation. Consequently, it is unnecessary to routinely identify the ureter.

- After a colostomy has been created, the pneumoperitoneum is reestablished and the colon is evaluated for torsion and hemostasis. Secondary trocars should be removed under direct vision.

- During takedown and closure of a Hartmann rectal turn-in, the anvil of the stapling device, inserted transanally, will help identify the rectal stump.

- If the intraperitoneal adhesions are extensive, it is usually good judgment to convert to an open procedure.

Surgical Technique

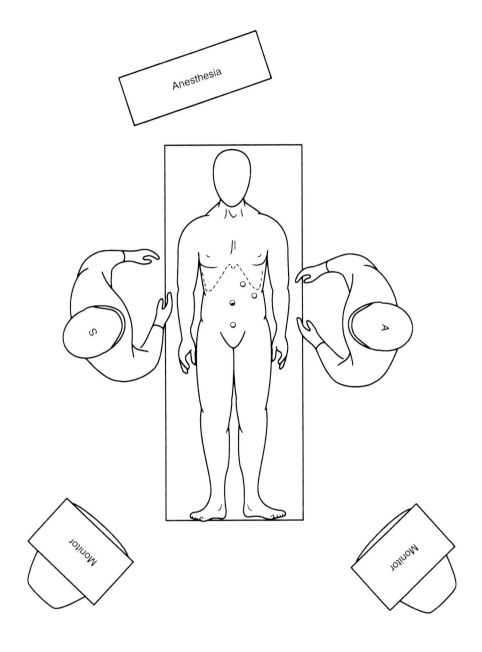

A   Operating room setup for a colostomy. The setup will be completely variable, depending on the anatomic site of the colostomy. Trocar placement for a colostomy will also vary, depending on the site that is clinically appropriate.

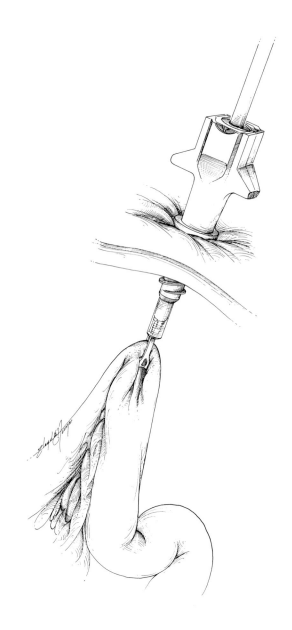

B   The appropriate segment of bowel is grasped by an anatomic bowel clamp and delivered through the trocar site.

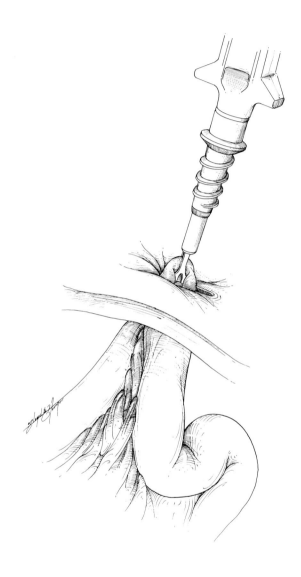

C By using the stoma site that was marked preoperatively, the bowel is delivered through the anterior abdominal wall.

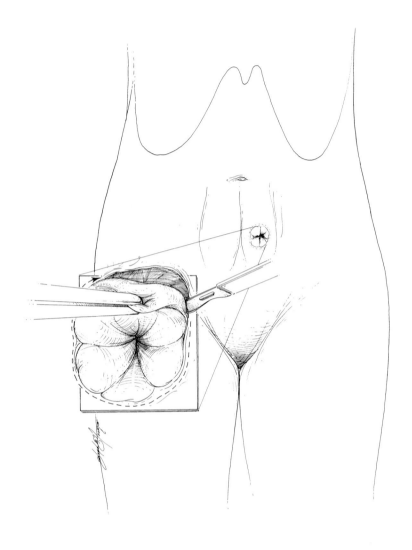

D   An incision is made at the mucocutaneous junction of the colostomy.

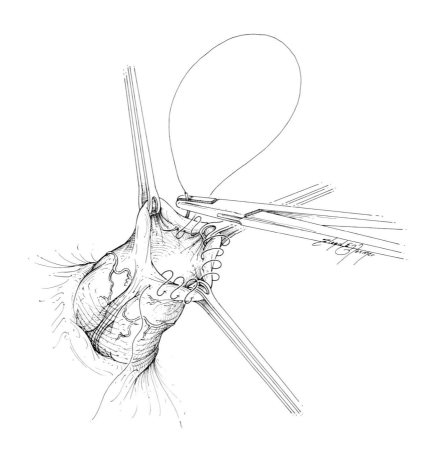

E   A purse-string suture is applied circumferentially after the colon is mobilized from the subcutaneous tissues.

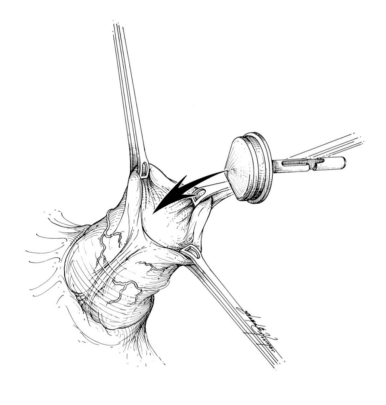

F   The anvil of the circular stapling device is inserted into the proximal colon.

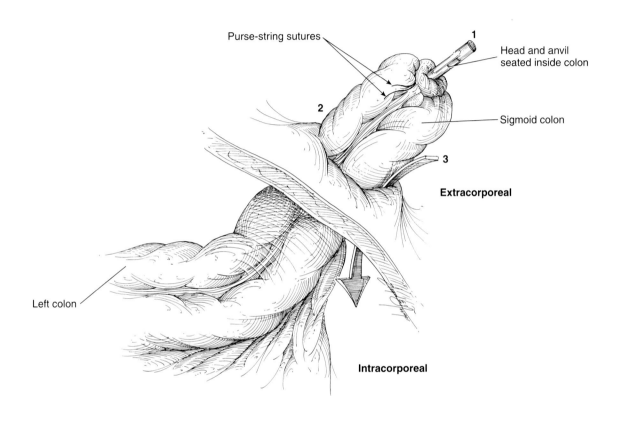

Purse-string sutures

Head and anvil
seated inside colon

Sigmoid colon

Extracorporeal

Left colon

Intracorporeal

G   The bowel, secured with purse-string sutures, is returned to the peritoneal cavity. A laparoscopic lysis of adhesions is performed if necessary.

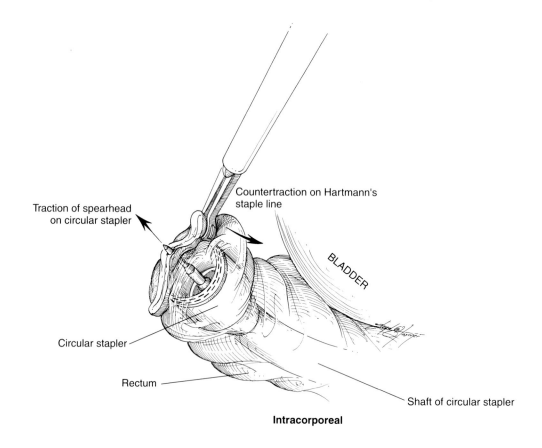

Traction of spearhead
on circular stapler

Countertraction on Hartmann's
staple line

BLADDER

Circular stapler

Rectum

Shaft of circular stapler

Intracorporeal

H The shaft of the stapler is placed transally and the anvil is extruded
through the staple line. A Babcock clamp is used to provide countertraction.

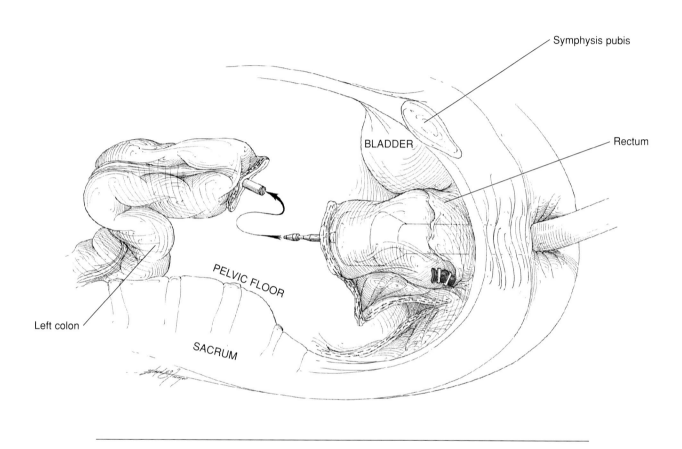

I   Cross-sectional view demonstrating insertion of the stapling device.

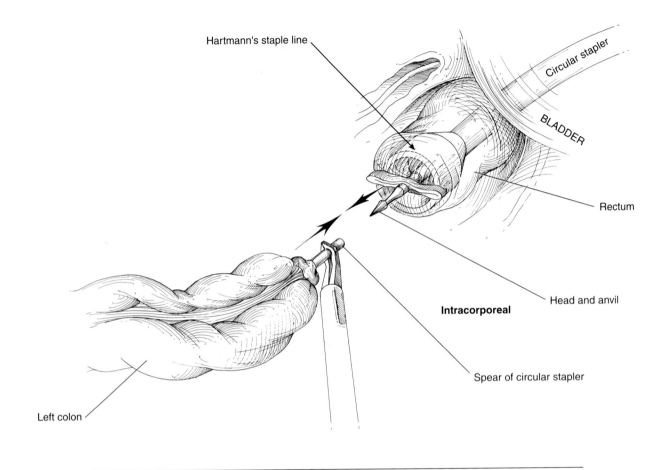

Hartmann's staple line

Circular stapler

BLADDER

Rectum

Head and anvil

Intracorporeal

Spear of circular stapler

Left colon

J   The surgeon orients the head and anvil with an instrument specifical-
ly devised for this purpose. An assistant stabilizes the shaft of the stapler to facilitate union.

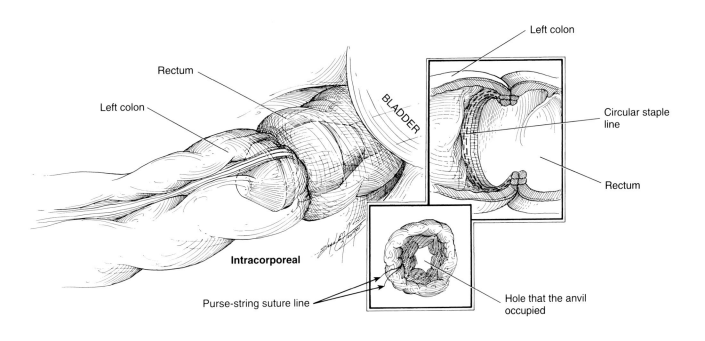

K The stapler is closed and fired. The "doughnuts" are examined for integrity of the anastomosis. *Upper inset:* Sagittal view of the completed anastomosis. *Lower inset:* Specimen made from circular cutter.

12

Rectopexy

Philip F. Caushaj · Moises Jacobs · Gustavo Plasencia

General Considerations

The laparoscopic approach for the treatment of rectal procidentia offers another modality in the surgeon's armamentarium. The issues regarding cost and the choice of abdominal versus transperineal procedures have not been resolved completely. However, the possibility of minimally invasive surgery for elderly high-risk patients is beneficial and may improve outcome. The same preoperative evaluation should occur for all patients. This is an excellent laparoscopic procedure for the tyro to master.

Preoperative Setup and Trocar Placement

The operating room setup is as for sigmoid resection and low anterior resection (Fig. *A*). Two television monitors are at the foot of the operating room table. The surgeon is positioned to the right of the patient while the assistant is to the left. The first trocar is inserted into the umbilicus and a diagnostic laparoscopy is performed. If there is no contraindication to proceeding with the laparoscopic technique, the secondary trocars are inserted in the left upper quadrant, left flank, and suprapubic region. The video camera is directed through the left upper quadrant trocar by the assistant.

Mobilization

The mobilization commences with the sigmoid colon. The assistant applies traction medially to the sigmoid by means of a Babcock clamp in the left flank trocar while the surgeon administers countertraction with a Babcock clamp through the umbilical trocar. The lateral peritoneal reflection is sharply incised with cautery scissors through the suprapubic trocar. Once these attachments are divided, the retroperitoneum is exposed. At this juncture, the left ureter is identified as previously described. We prefer to identify the pulsations of the iliac artery, and using this anatomic landmark, locate the ureter.

The assistant places traction directly on the mesentery through the left flank trocar and the surgeon uses the umbilical trocar. This traction causes the inferior mesenteric vessels to become taut and thus easily identified. The surgeon scores the peritoneum distal to the inferior mesenteric vessels and the retrorectal space is entered (Fig. 12-1). Anterior traction is applied to the rectum by the assistant by means of a Babcock clamp in the left flank trocar, while the surgeon applies additional anterior traction through the suprapubic trocar. A cautery spatula is inserted through the suprapubic trocar, and with blunt and sharp dissection the rectum is freed to the

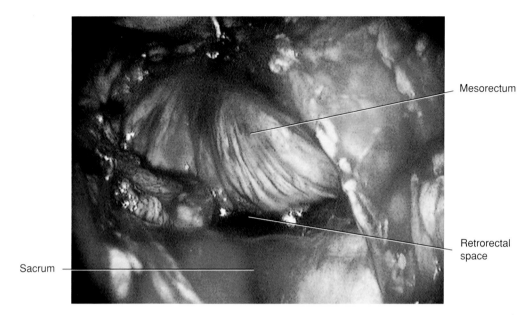

Mesorectum

Retrorectal
space

Sacrum

Fig. 12-1. Superior dissection of the retroperitoneum exposes the sacrum during rectopexy.

level of the levator ani muscles. This includes sharp division of Waldeyer's fascia.

Proximally, the surgeon and assistant expose the promontory of the sacrum using blunt dissection. The sacral promontory is initially located by direct palpation with the dissecting instruments. With blunt dissection the fibrous layer of the sacrum is mobilized until the bony sacrum is visualized. We recommend gentle technique in the area of the sacral promontory—hemorrhage from the presacral vessels can be copious and alarming. Once the middle of the sacral promontory is cleared, dissection is continued several centimeters into the sacral hollow (Fig. 12-2).

It is important for the surgeon and assistant to reduce the procidentia by applying traction superiorly through Babcock clamps in the umbilical and left flank trocars, respectively. A measure of caution dictates examination of the rectum by an unscrubbed but gloved assistant to ensure complete reduction.

At this point, a 6 by 4 cm piece of Prolene mesh (Vicryl) is placed via the suprapubic trocar into the peritoneal cavity (Fig. 12-3). A hernia stapling device is inserted through the suprapubic trocar and two parallel rows of staples are placed in the midline of the mesh, securing the mesh to the sacrum (Fig. 12-3). The mesh now has a medial and lateral unattached wing (Fig. 12-4); these wings are draped over the rectum on both sides. It is imperative that the assistant continue traction to the rectum in an anterior

Pelvis

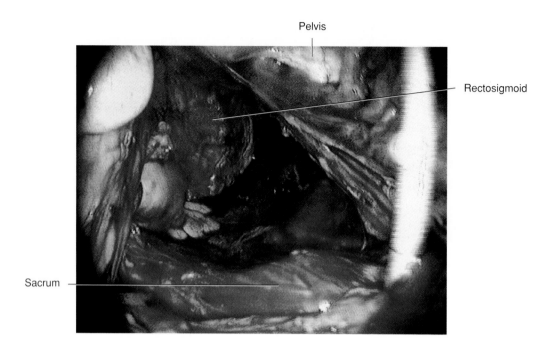

Rectosigmoid

Sacrum

Fig. 12-2. Mobilization of the rectosigmoid in a view deep into the pelvis.

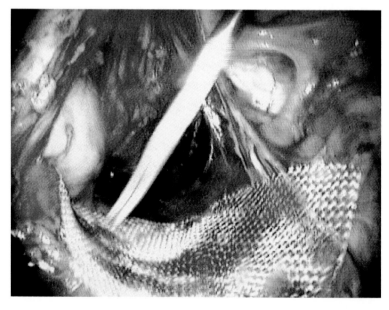

Fig. 12-3. Vicryl mesh is delivered intraperitoneally into the sacral hollow.

and superior direction to maintain reduction of the procidentia. The wings of the mesh are now secured to the rectum, encompassing a 270-degree circumference of the rectum (Fig. 12-5). This allows the anterior surface of the rectum to be unconstricted.

The mesh may be secured to the rectum either with the use of a hernia stapler or by laparoscopic suturing (see Fig. 12-5). We prefer to use the stapling device; however, we do not attempt to penetrate the rectum full-

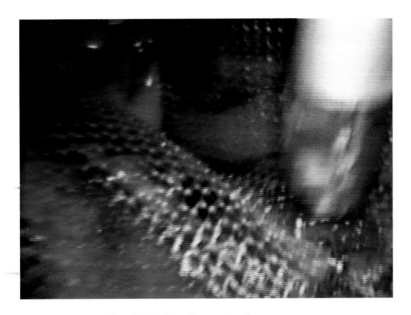

Fig. 12-4. Stapling into the sacrum.

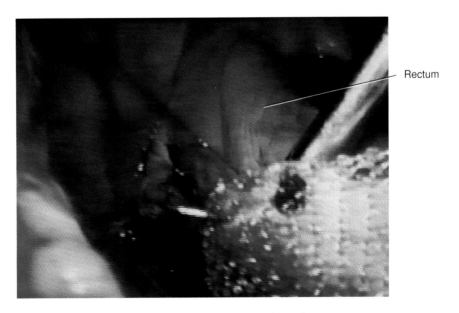

Rectum

Fig. 12-5. Suturing of the Vicryl mesh.

thickness. Indeed, if the stapler is used, the staples are placed in the fat of the rectum and the mesentery (Fig. 12-6).

At the completion of the procedure we again examine the rectum to ensure that the procidentia has been reduced and perform rigid proctosigmoidoscopy to ensure that the staples have not penetrated the rectum full-thickness. The secondary trocars are removed under direct vision and the incisions are closed (Fig. 12-7).

Rectum ———

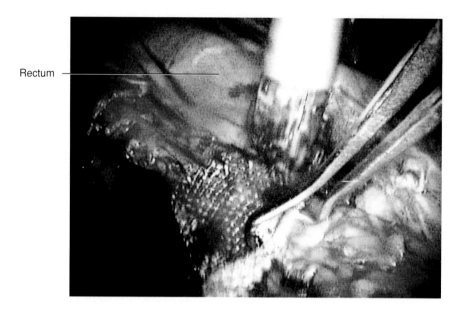

Fig. 12-6. A staple is placed into the rectum while the rectum is held under tension.

Rectum ———

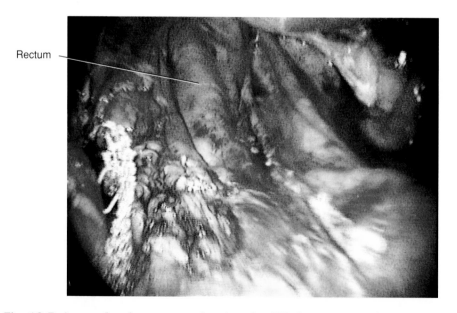

Fig. 12-7. A completed rectopexy showing the 270-degree wrap of Vicryl mesh around the rectum (compare Fig. *L*, p. 229).

Clinical Caveats

- It is essential to maintain appropriate tension on the bowel so that the rectal procidentia is completely reduced. This is particularly important when performing a laparoscopic rectopexy.

- If hemorrhage is encountered from the presacral veins, it may be necessary to employ one of the following techniques approached laparoscopically to occlude the hemorrhage: direct tamponade by a hernia staple into the sacrum, occlusion by hernia staple and Surgicel applied directly to the sacrum, or laparoscopic placement of a sterile thumb tack to the sacrum.

- At the termination of the procedure, the anus should be reexamined to be certain that the procidentia has been reduced.

Surgical Technique

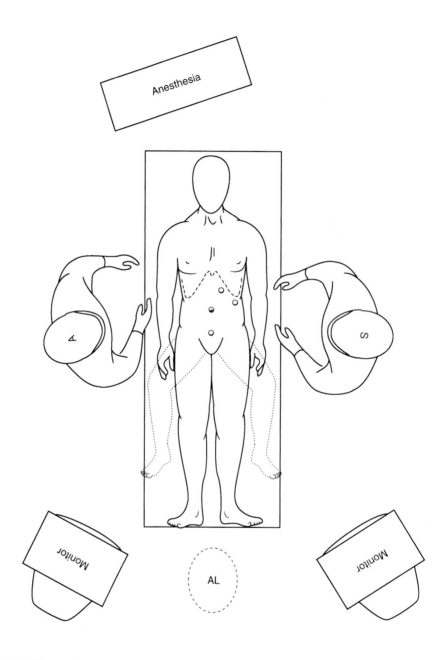

A Operating room setup for rectopexy. *S,* surgeon; *A,* assistant, *AL,* alternative location for assistant. Note suggested trocar placement.

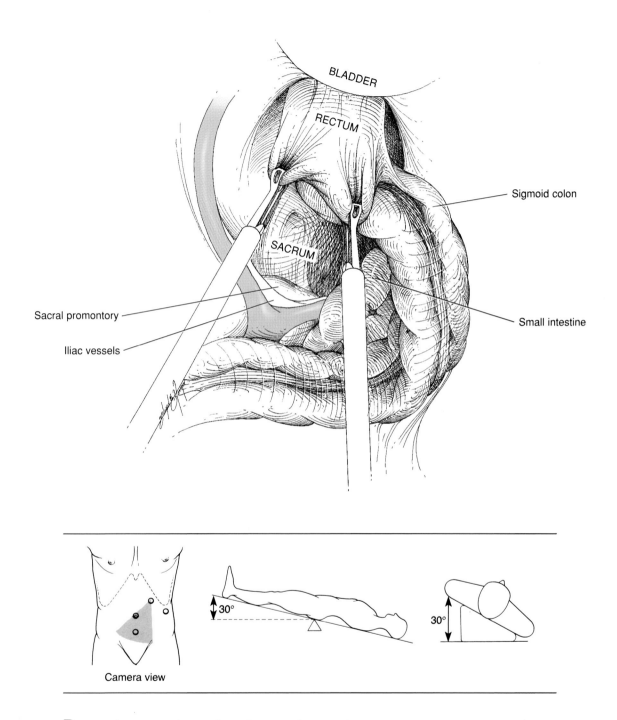

B   Reduction of rectal prolapse. This is important to prevent recurrence.

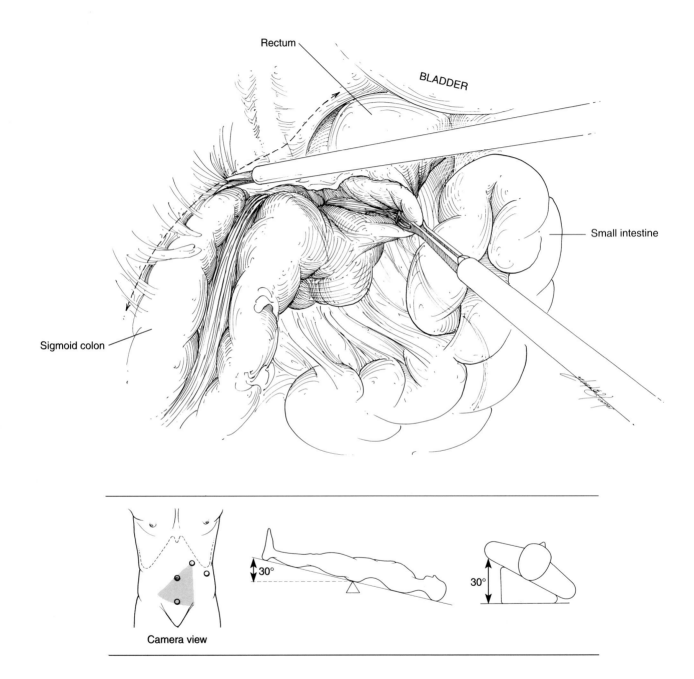

Rectum

BLADDER

Small intestine

Sigmoid colon

Camera view

30°

30°

C Mobilization of the sigmoid colon by incising the left peritoneal reflection.

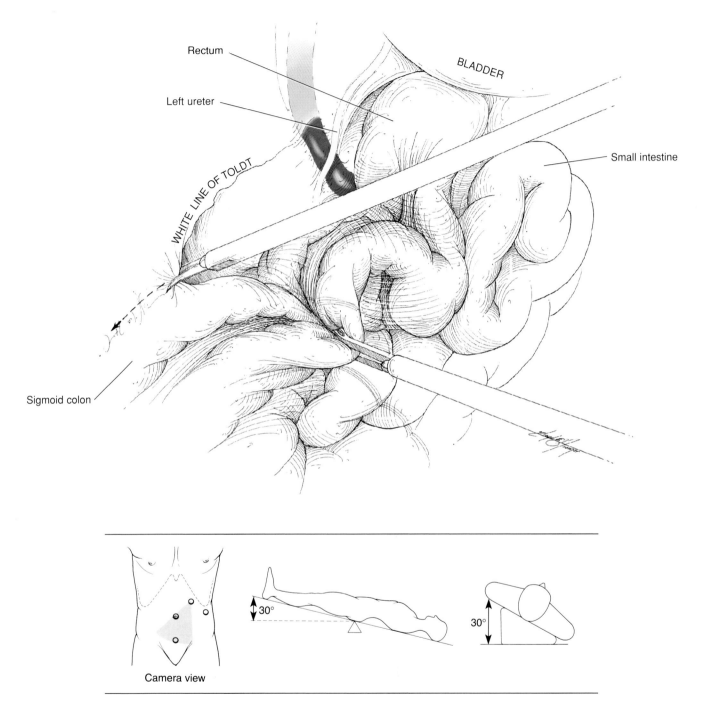

Rectum

Left ureter

BLADDER

WHITE LINE OF TOLDT

Small intestine

Sigmoid colon

Camera view

30°

30°

D   It is essential to identify the left ureter before vascular ligation.

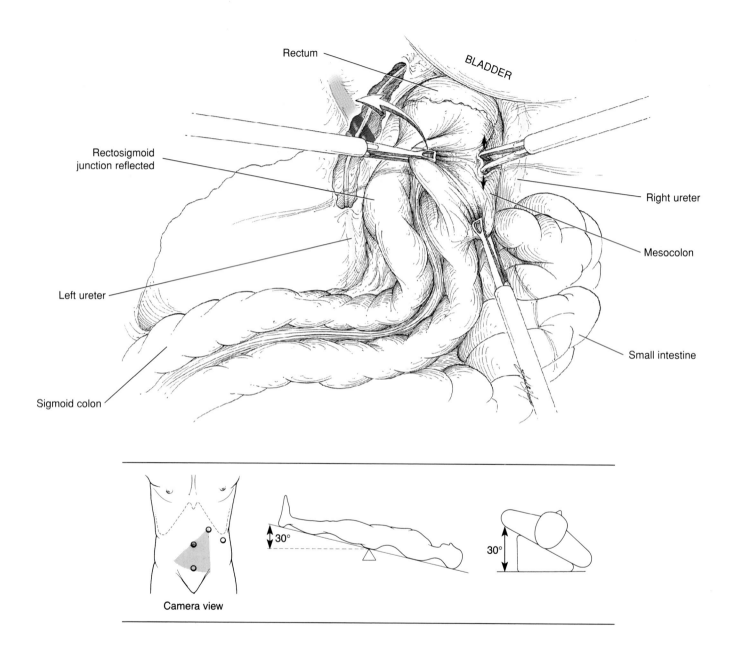

Rectum

BLADDER

Rectosigmoid
junction reflected

Right ureter

Mesocolon

Left ureter

Small intestine

Sigmoid colon

Camera view

30°

30°

E   Incision of the right iliac fossa at the base of the mesosigmoid to completely develop the plane into the retrorectal space.

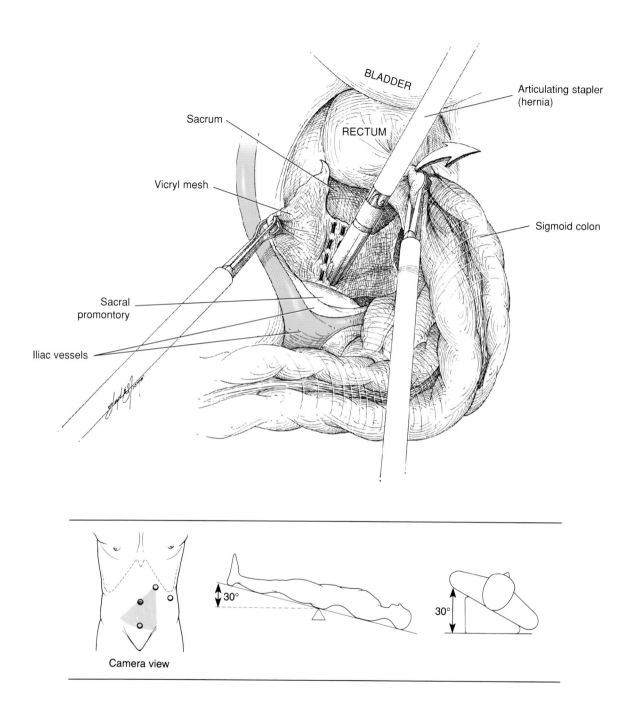

F   Once adequate mobilization to the levator ani is performed, the Vicryl mesh is stapled to the sacrum.

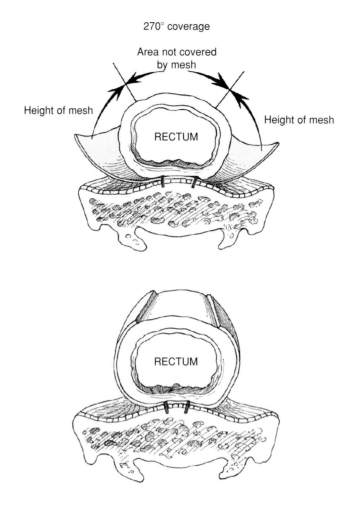

G *Top,* Cross-sectional view of mesh secured to the sacral promontory and rectum. *Bottom,* When the mesh is secured to the rectum, it is important to maintain superior traction on the rectum so that prolapse does not recur.

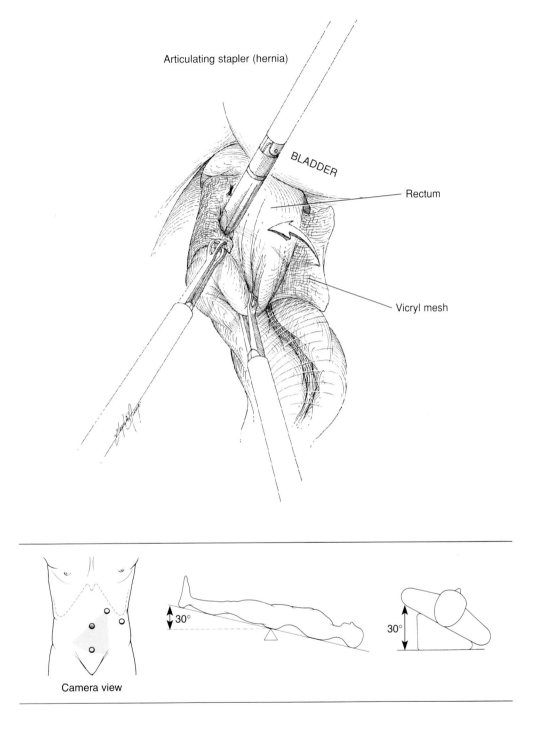

H   The Vicryl mesh can be secured with staples or sutured. If staplers are used, it is important to ensure that the staples are not full-thickness.

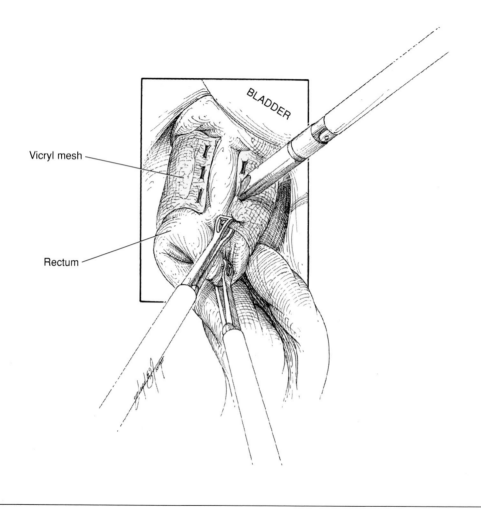

I   Completed 270-degree wrap of the rectum with Vicryl mesh.

Index